PROBLEM PERIODS:
Causes, Symptoms and Relief
Dr. Caroline Shreeve

GW00504170

Piccadilly Press · London

Phototypeset by Goodfellow & Egan, Cambridge
Printed and bound by Bath Press, Bath
for the publishers, Piccadilly Press Ltd.,
5 Castle Road, London NW1 8PR

A catalogue record for this book is available from the
British Library

ISBN: 1 85340 295 8

Dr Caroline Shreeve lives in East Sussex. She is a very
experienced doctor. She is the author of many books,
mainly on women's health. This is her first book for
Piccadilly Press.

CONTENTS

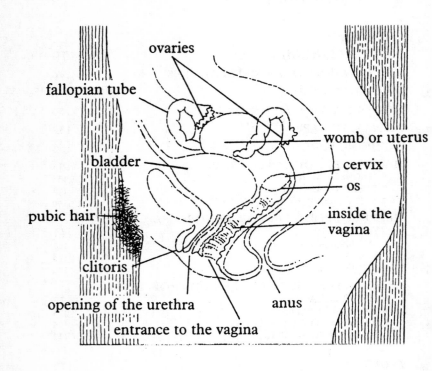

ovaries

fallopian tube

bladder

pubic hair

clitoris

opening of the urethra

entrance to the vagina

womb or uterus

cervix

os

inside the vagina

anus

Chapter One

Normal Menstruation

Period problems can make you feel distressed and isolated, especially when investigations prove negative or your GP recommends letting nature take her course, then inexplicably writes out a prescription!

The womb and menstrual cycle are the physical/functional tip of a highly emotive iceberg; this is self-evident when you see how lives can be wrecked by rape, and how infertility can destroy a woman's self-esteem. But it's important to remember their central rôle in our lives, even those of us who lack partners and/or the wish to have children, if we're to understand how profoundly emotional and psychological factors can affect our periods.

It's certainly easy to misinterpret normal variations and minor menstrual problems. Up to middle age, you may worry unnecessarily about light, heavy or irregular periods (which may need checking if they persist, but are rarely serious). Later, you may pass off post-menopausal bleeding (the resumption of bleeding a year or so after your final period), as your body's final fling. Individual differences can also cause concern: our cycle length; how many days we bleed and how much blood we lose; are all affected by our makeup, lifestyle and environment as, too, are our perception of, and response to, pain and other symptoms.

WHAT IS 'NORMAL?'

'Normal values' quoted in textbooks of physiology are based on averages obtained from large numbers of healthy people. Doctors have to work within agreed guidelines like anyone else, and acceptable ranges are usually wide. Familiar examples are pulse rate and blood pressure. The 'average' heart beats between about seventy and eighty times per minute at rest; but a couch potato's pulse may well bomb along considerably faster, while a sportsman or woman in training is likely to have a pulse of 60 beats/minute or lower. Both count as normal.

Again, very few healthy people maintain a standard blood pressure (BP) of 120/80 millimeters of mercury (mm. Hg), the units used to measure this body function, and which you can see in the glass mercury column when an old-fashioned blood pressure cuff is used. A few minutes linked to an electronic sphygnomanometer illustrates that the slightest stress involved in watching your level on an LCD screen can push up your reading by 20 mm. Hg or more.

Similarly, individual menstrual cycles vary greatly, and our personal pattern can change from month to month. Cycles can range from 13 to 50 days in length, and are still considered normal. In fact a study carried out in 1977 revealed that only 12.4% of women (80 in every 500), actually have a standard 28 day cycle, making this length the commonest by the merest whisker.

PAIN CAN BE NORMAL

Pain is tissue-talk – the voice of the body or one of its organs speaking a primitive language we can all understand but which we mostly try to stifle. Listening to the message *before* reaching for pain-killers, can reduce stress and distress, since it often originates from a normal, rather than an abnormal, source.

Labour and delivery have to be the most natural processes ever, yet you have only to compare the largest diameter of a full-term infant's head (about 13.5 cms./5.5 ins. from chin to crown), with that of the fully dilated cervix (about 10 cms/4 ins.) or the narrowest portion of the birth canal (10 cms.

4 ins.+), to understand the pain birth can cause. Alternatively, the next time you remove a tampon, imagine that its upper end is attached to a large melon inside your womb, which you're going to have to drag down through your slightly widened cervix.

MUSCULAR SPASM = PAIN

Delivery is brought about by the squeezing actions of the heftily muscular womb walls, which push the infant along, and finally out of, the birth canal. Contractions build up as more force is required, and hurt like all muscular spasm because they nip blood vessels, restricting the flow of blood. This deprives the tissues of oxygen and permits toxic chemical by-products (metabolites) such as lactic acid, to accumulate, stimulating nearby pain-sensitive nerve endings.

Other forms of painful muscular spasm include: renal colic involving the ureters – tubes connecting kidneys and bladder; gall bladder (biliary) colic; bladder and urethral (urinary outlet tube) spasm, common in cystitis, and the agonising gastric and abdominal cramps accompanying vomiting and diarrhoea during a food-poisoning attack.

During a period, the womb walls contract similarly to expel the waste contents into the vagina.

Period pains are, therefore, natural and not in the least dangerous, and easier than most other forms of muscular spasm to relieve.

HOW MUCH DOES MENSTRUATION BOTHER OTHER WOMEN?

We certainly have plenty of time to get used to menstrual pain and trivial irregularities. A woman with average twenty-eight-day cycles that start at the age of 12, end when she's 50, and pause only for two full term pregnancies and two six week periods of breast-feeding, including false periods on the Pill, tots up around 470 periods!

Our attitude to problem periods has improved since the fifties when menstruation was still viewed with Victorian distaste, and information about it practically non-existent. Periods are now discussed openly, and more and more women forget about them entirely while they remain troublefree, except with respect to contraception or pregnancy.

Nothing could delight us when we're frantic about an overdue period, as much as that first show of blood or twinge of pelvic cramp; nor anything distress us more, if we're trying to conceive. However, problem periods still have great nuisance potential, and identifying likely causes can help avoid unnecessary discomfort and concern.

Nagging period fears can escalate into cancer or AIDS phobias when you're stressed, so it's equally useful to be able to distinguish between minor ailments that are best left alone or treated with natural remedies; and more serious ones requiring medical advice. First, a few facts about the organs involved, and the hormones that control them.

THE MENSTRUAL CYCLE

Menstrual bleeding has been called 'the tears of a disappointed uterus'. Though coy by today's tastes, the notion is apt. The cycle *is* designed to prepare a biologically suitable environment for the development of a fertilized egg; and if the egg is not fertilized, the carefully orchestrated preparations that take place between the last day of a period and ovulation are entirely wasted. Tennyson was right to call Nature 'red in tooth and claw' (*In Memorium*).

Ovulation means the discharge of a ripe egg (ovum) from one or other ovary, into the nearby Fallopian tubes – the long, hollow arms coming off the right and left sides of the top of the uterus. Each tube ends in a cup with finger-like fronds or fimbria, which help direct the egg into the tube's interior where it can be fertilized by a sperm.

Whether or not this happens, the egg passes down into the womb, its passage aided by tiny hairs or cilia on the tube's lining that waft it in the right direction. A fertilized egg burrows into the womb's vascular wall and starts 'dividing and multiplying' into an embryo. An unfertilized egg shrivels up and leaves the body in the menstrual blood.

The hormones regulating the menstrual cycle's every step, are secreted by endocrine glands controlled by the master pituitary gland in the centre of the brain which, in turn, is governed by the hypothalamus. This highly specialised area of grey matter below the midbrain is the site of our thermostat and appestat (temperature and appetite) controls. It also has close links with the adrenal glands responsible for the fright, flight and fight stress responses, and is a neurological focus for the integration and control of moods and emotions.

Influenced by follicle stimulating hormone (FSH) from the pituitary, unripe eggs in the ovaries mature into fluid-filled blisters called ovarian or Graafian follicles. These release oestrogen to develop and thicken the womb lining, aid the passage of sperm and ova along the Fallopian tube, and modify the chemical composition, texture and acidity of the cervical mucus to encourage sperm to enter. (Acidity depends on the number of free, electrically-charged hydrogen atoms present, a factor expressed as a solution's pH. With seven being neutral, higher values represent alkalinity and lower values, acidity).

Of the 100 or so ovarian follicles that ripen every cycle, one only – the ripest of all – reaches the surface of the ovary and continues to develop, in some cases to the size of a cherry. At ovulation, the outer coating of the follicle has to burst to release the egg within; and if the follicle is a large one, this can cause a mild ache or a sharpish twinge in the groin or lower tummy.

About one in ten women experience this discomfort, called Mittelschmerz (German, meaning 'middle of the month'), and a few also have a slight ovulatory bleed as well. This is harmless, and caused by the complex hormonal changes taking place.

Normally, the remaining follicles shrink back into the substance of the ovary and disappear. Occasionally, one continues to grow into a fluid-filled sac or cyst, containing either watery tissue fluid or a fatty liquid and, in some cases, fragments of hair and teeth as well. (The latter develop from cells embryologists call pluripotential. As their name suggests, these cells are potentially capable of growing into almost any type of tissue).

Most cysts arising from follicles are benign (non-cancerous), but they can grow larger than a newborn baby's head. Symptoms include discomfort, a swollen tummy, and maybe urinary or bowel disturbances as well, due to pressure.

One of several things can happen. Single and/or small cysts can disappear of their own accord; or discomfort may lead to their discovery and surgical removal. More seriously, they can twist on their stalk (known medically as 'torsion'), nipping their own blood supply and causing severe abdominal pain; or rupture and discharge their contents (plus blood) into the abdominal cavity (also painful). Alternatively, they can interfere with the blood supply to another abdominal or pelvic organ such as an ovary, loop of bowel or the bladder, a condition also requiring emergency surgery.

Polycystic ovaries, which cause irregular bleeding, are discussed in Chapter 5.

Influenced by luteinising hormone (LH) from the pituitary gland, the newly-vacated Graafian follicle or corpus luteum (Latin for 'yellow body', it does have a faintly yellow colour) releases progesterone, which further thickens and softens the womb lining. At the time of ovulation, this lining, also called the endometrium, is thick, soft and spongy, highly vascular and chock-full of special nutrients ready and waiting in small, cellular sacs.

When Professor David Horrobin (UK and Canada) experimented with taking LH which he believed to be partially responsible for the premenstrual syndrome (PMS), he suffered from fluid retention, bloating, weight gain, breast tenderness and irritability – all major signs of the condition (see Chapter 7). This brave experiment (at least psychosociologically if not physiologically!), led to the discovery of the key role of essential fatty acid GLA, and its application to the treatment of PMS. More about this in Chapter 8.

Progesterone levels start to fall around the 22nd day. Around day 25–27 in a 28 day cycle, the corpus luteum shrivels, oestrogen and progesterone levels continue to fall, and the uterine blood vessels clamp down under the influence of progesterone, reducing the oxygen and nutrient supply to the womb lining, which then begins to disintegrate, fold over on itself and finally come away from the womb wall. The womb walls contract in response to the tissue and blood within. For 4–5 days, red blood cells and womb lining tissue mixed with cellular secretions are discharged from the vagina as period blood.

The first day on which the bleeding starts is day one of the next menstrual cycle.

WHAT AFFECTS THE CYCLE?

1. DIET
This must in many ways affect hormone production, the development of cells, the health and

functional ability of organ linings and their resistance to infection and other diseases; and, of course, fertility. Taking extreme examples: the eating disorder anorexia nervosa halts menstruation when the body weight has fallen below a certain critical level; while obesity, due either to inborn errors of metabolism or simply comfort bingeing on junk foods, can hamper concentration.

Specific Nutrient Deficiencies e.g. of *vitamin E*, normally obtained from wheat germ, wholegrain cereals, eggs, green leafy vegetables and plant and grain cooking oils, can also affect fertility. Our vitamin E requirement increases if we take the Pill or other synthetic hormones, drink chlorinated tap water, or eat large amounts of polyunsaturated fats.

Zinc from red meat and offal, wheat germ, brewer's yeast, pumpkin seeds and ground mustard, is necessary for the normal growth of the reproductive organs. You need more of this mineral if you drink heavily, are diabetic, or take supplements of vitamin B6 (pyridoxine). Supplementary zinc, in turn, increases your need for beta carotene (pro-vitamin A), and helps to relieve certain forms of depressive illness (see PMS, Chapter 7).

2. THE PILL

The combined oestrogen-progestogen Pill, e.g. Mercilon, Ovranette, works by imitating the feedback effect of the natural hormones on the pituitary and hypothalamus. This prevents the release of FSH and LH, needed for the development of a mature Graafian follicle, and also for ovulation. Synthetic combined Pill hormones also affect the womb's endometrial lining, the quality of the cervical mucus, and the 'friendliness' of the Fallopian tubes to travelling sperm. 'False' periods occur with combined Pills allowing pill-free days between packs when stopping oestrogen brings on a withdrawal bleed; but not with the every day combined Pill, which allows no such gap.

Progestogen-only oral contraceptives e.g. Femulen, Micronor, also work by reducing the receptivity of the womb, cervix and tubes to sperm. They can suppress ovulation completely in some women, in which case you would not bleed at all; other users go on ovulating and bleeding as usual. The progestogen-only Pill sometimes causes irregular blood loss, but it suits large numbers of many women (e.g. smokers over 35) unable to take the combined variety.

Ovulation can take several months to return after stopping the Pill, but some women conceive almost at once.

3. MENTAL STRESS

This can bring periods to a halt temporarily through its direct effect on hypothalmus. Common factors having this effect include relationship problems, bereavement, redundancy, divorce and moving house.

Foreign holidays (which, like emigrating, can cause culture shock), are also sometimes responsible. Cases have been reported of au pair girls not menstruating for up to six months after starting work in a new country.

4. PHYSICAL STRESS

This may act similarly; periods can stop after a serious accident or during convalescence, and prolonged chronic stress due to a physically demanding job, being a workaholic or simply working long hours in combination with crash dieting and, perhaps, relationship difficulties, can have the same result.

5. PHEROMONES

These are molecular particles released by bodily areas, and capable of carrying messages of a person's state of health and mind, and of sexual metabolism. Falling in love may be mediated by pheromones without our being aware of it; sexual chemistry is thought probably to be explained by pheromones, although this is unfortunate when person A's instinctive attraction towards person B's 'molecular activators' is unreciprocated. Possibly love spells and potions of old worked on the pheromone principle, especially aromatherapy essences such as rose, sandalwood and ylang ylang, all potent aphrodisiacs. The idea has been put forward that such oils worked by modifying the would-be attractor's 'sublime odour', so that their projected attractee was automatically drawn to them regardless of their own chemical odour conformation.

Dogs are demonstrably able to pick up their mistress's cyclical state just by sniffing. With nasal powers ten thousand times stronger than man's, they have little difficulty in assimilating and digesting mentally whether 'She' is especially vulnerable at a particular time, e.g. when premenstrual or menstruating; and some, depending on their temperament and relationship with their owner, will take advantage of this knowledge.

This is especially evident in the case of 'whole' (non-castrated) males, who like to establish themselves as pack leader; this can lead to relationship problems when the woman owner is equally determined to keep her canine friend one step behind! (The solution is usually learning to be more assertive, and detracting from the dog's often sublimely high opinion of himself as protector and boss – in the kindest possible way, naturally).

Pheromones are also thought to be responsible for the synchrony women's cycles undergo when they live together in a group; within months, their periods coincide more or less closely, a fact strenuously denied in the past by keepers of convents and hostels.

WHAT ABOUT LEGENDARY INFLUENCES?

The tidal pull of the moon was, and often still is, believed to influence menstrual blood flow. After all, it is the 28 day lunar month, not the Gregorian calendar month, with which the 'standard' cycle concurs.

Astrologers and occultists are not the only groups of people inclined to this view. Studies in Europe and America have shown that periods tend to be affected by the tides, strongly under lunar control, the Earth's oceans and seas being the macrocosmic equivalent of microcosmic blood, lymph and tissue fluid – not to mention fluid hormonal secretions. Since the phases of the moon regulate tidal forces, say exponents of this idea, isn't it logical to suppose they similarly affect the 'tides' in the human body, too (although I've never met a doctor who supports the idea).

Claude Bernard[1] was the first to describe our internal environment, which he referred to as 'le milieu interieur'. All forces in the macrocosm

15

(surrounding universe and planet Earth) are replicated in miniature in man's person, which he called the microcosm. Much of our understanding of the interrelationship and interdependence of bodily processes and also of homoeostasis – the condition of fully integrated function – owes much to Bernard's genius.

TWO COMMON WORRIES

1. SEX DURING PERIODS

The health risks are minimal, although popularly supposed to be non-existent. I will summarise an answer to a recent question on this topic from a lecturer in Obstetrics and Gynaecology to a GP in a medical journal.

Firstly, he doesn't believe there is any increased risk of developing cervical cancer although a link between cancer and sex during menstruation has been considered in this context before. He says that some women with this disease do secrete smaller amounts of a protective enzyme called alpha-1-antitrypsin in their cervical fluid than non-sufferers, thus having less resistance to 'biological insults', i.e. potentially harmful factors,

[1](1813–78), Professor of Physiology at the Sorbonne, Paris and of Medicine at the College de France, still regarded as the greatest physiologist of all time.

16

such as sperm. But he hastens to add that there is no evidence that such decreased immunity is commoner during menstruation.

The theoretical objections this expert cites, centre mainly on the increased blood supply to the womb and vagina that typifies menstrual periods; one is that the flow may suddenly increase, as the womb's arteries and veins dilate and become congested with blood, as they always do when sexual excitement mounts.

Two other theoretical possibilities include damage to the more vascular and easily-damaged vagina from the penis; and the waves of uterine muscular contraction during orgasm, causing the retrograde muscular contraction that can lead to endometriosis (please see Chapter 3).

However, he does say that a chronic infection of either partner's reproductive organs could (conceivably) either flare up or give rise to salpingitis (inflamed and damaged Fallopian tubes); and adds that menstruation alone could do this, even without the intercourse factor. A condom, Dutch cap or some other barrier method would offer protection; but there is no need for this in healthy couples, who ought not to be discouraged from love making during a period, especially as some women's libido is higher at that time of the month.

Jewish women are forbidden to have intercourse during menstruation and for seven days afterwards. This so-called safe period, on the other hand, constitutes the only contraceptive method presently permitted by the Roman Catholic Church. As a family-planning technique it is less than reliable – the risks of getting pregnant then are minimal, not non-existent. But in its favour, menstrual intercourse is better for both partners, psychologically and emotionally, than coitus interruptus (man withdraws before climax) or coitus interfemoris (man ejaculates between his partner's thighs).

2. SWIMMING DURING PERIODS

Swimming and other common forms of exercise are safe when you are menstruating. Benefits include a boost when you're feeling depressed or out of sorts, and relief from pelvic and back pain. Physical activity, especially the aerobic sort that increases pulse and makes you breathe harder, speeds up the circulation and gets the blood moving in the pelvic arteries and veins where painful congestion occurs. It can also improve bowel movements, combating the sluggishness and constipation that can aggravate congestion and uterine spasm.

Avoid bathing in icy water if tummy cramps bother you – extreme cold could bring on an attack. By the same token, avoid sitting around in a wet bikini or bathing costume for hours – common sense is vital for coping with problem periods! And avoid, for example, gymnastics, other risky sports and strenuous long distance running or jogging if you get dizzy, faint or sick during periods. Instead, get your doctor to check your blood for iron deficiency anaemia, particularly if your periods are heavy, and take a daily iron supplement.

BENIGN COITAL HEADACHE

It is tempting to add a word about this distressing complaint in *Problem Periods*, although it is not directly related to menstruation and it affects both sexes. It was first described as a distinct form of headache associated with sexual intercourse in a publication by Dr. K Kritz as recently as 1970, although headache linked to sexual excitement has been recognised since the time of Hippocrates of Cos (around 400 BC).

The condition is called benign because it is not underpinned by a serious underlying disease; yet the vascular headache that pounds and throbs in time with your heartbeat, produces the most agonising pain. Speech and movement may become impossible, some victims faint or go into shock, and many report afterwards that they thought they were dying of a sudden brain tumour or haemorrhage. The course of the condition is largely unpredictable; some people have one or two attacks that are never repeated, while others suffer sporadically for months or years at times of mounting sexual excitement.

A fourteen year follow-up study of 24 men and eight women, carried out from 1978 to 1991 at the University Hospital of Arhus in Denmark by Drs. John Ustergard and Morten Kraft, showed that sufferers from benign coital headache are characteristically vulnerable at certain times and not at all at others (half the patients had had a recurrence after an interval of up to ten years); and that the risks of recurrent clusters of disabling head pain were far greater in those who also suffered from tension headaches or migraine.

A cause for recurrent attacks not mentioned in this paper in the British Medical Journal, is the hypertensive crisis or 'cheese effect' that can befall anyone taking a course of certain antidepressants,[1] if they eat forbidden tyramine-rich foods or drinks, producing a severe rise in blood pressure. Examples are stale foods, especially rancid offal and meat, mature cheese, broad bean pods, tinned green figs, pickled herrings (rollmops), flavoured textured vegetable protein (often called PHP, a substitute for proper meat), Oxo, Bovril, Marmite and Chianti wine.

[1] le monoamine oxidase inhibitor (MAOI) antidepressants e.g. tranylcypromine – Parnate, Parstelin or plenylzine-Nardil.

A host of drugs including adrenaline, opiate pain-killers such as codeine and morphine, appetite suppressant fenfluramine (Ponderax – prescribed for slimmers), tricyclic antidepressants e.g. clomipramine (Anafranil), amoxapine (Asendis), and cold remedies and decongestants containing ephedrine or pseudoephedrine (Sinutab, Sudafed, Day Nurse, Night Nurse) or phenyl-propanolamine (Dimotapp LA, Eskornade, Contac 400) *and many others* can also trigger a reaction.

Chapter Two

YOUR FIRST PERIOD

The first period is called the menarche (men-ark-ee), and its arrival can be stressful, because of the hormonal changes during and preceding it, the symptoms you can experience, and the importance schoolgirls attach to 'who has and who hasn't yet started...'.

WHEN DO MOST GIRLS START?

More than eighty per cent of girls start menstruating between the ages of 13 and 14, 95% start between 11 and 15, and the remainder at either end of this age range, start between 10 and 11, or 15 and 16.[1] These figures especially interest clinical environmentalists and nutritionists, who believe that the earlier start of menstruation compared with 30 years ago reflects improved diet and living standards.

[1] Ruth Cochrane, Senior Registrar in Obstetrics and Gynaecology, St Mary's Hospital, London, in her feature on *The Menarche* in *The Practitioner*, May 1993.

What Causes the Menarche?

The sequence of events leading up to the menarche, starts with the release of hormones from the hypothalamus which in turn stimulate the pituitary gland to secrete FSH (see Chapter 1) to ripen the ovarian follicles. Ovulation occurs as described earlier, under the influence of LH from the pituitary, and the menstrual cycle is underway.

This all sounds very sudden, but we know from ultrasound studies that the egg follicles in the ovary develop throughout childhood. The menarche is simply the culmination of rising oestrogen levels which bring about puberty – sexual development which can start as early as nine or ten, and includes the appearance of secondary sexual characteristics, i.e. breasts; pubic and other body hair; changes in shape and size of vaginal lips (labia), clitoris and pelvic bone structure; altered voice timbre; and the definition of a waist with redistributed body fat, e.g. less on tummy, more on hips, thighs and upper arms.

Delayed Puberty

This means a lack of the necessary changes leading up to that period in life when it becomes possible to father or conceive a child. The cause can sometimes be traced to a failure of one of the links between the brain and endocrine (hormone secreting) glands, since the whole process of puberty depends on the maturation of the hypothalamus (see Chapter 1), which influences the adrenal glands and the ovaries via the pituitary gland.

Here we come back to pheromones, which are believed to be responsible for the effects of the hypothalamus on sex hormone production. The ability of FSH and LH to stimulate the ovaries is enhanced by oestrogens made in layers of fat below the skin from chemical precursors provided by the adrenals. Thus body weight and body fat directly affect puberty, the menarche occurring on average at around 47 kg (7.5 stone), although the range is wide.

We all feature some aspects of the opposite sex; and androgens (male hormones) from the outer layer or cortex of the adrenal glands are responsible for the growth spurt which peaks about 11 months before the menarche, and the appearance of secondary sexual characteristics such as a change in voice timbre, and the growth of underarm and pubic hair. (Pubic hair usually starts to grow, along with the genitals, after the breasts have shown signs of enlarging, usually around the age of 11. The normal range for the start of breast development is between 9–13 years, and it takes around five years to complete). Underarm hair may start to grow before or after the menarche.

DELAYED MENARCHE

This means failure to menstruate by the age of 18. Sometimes, menstruation starts spontaneously; in other cases, the cause can be traced to a glandular problem in the areas mentioned above in connection with delayed puberty. But when secondary sexual characteristics have developed normally, the cause may be imperfect formation (atresia) of the vagina or cervix, leading to retention of menstrual blood flow – a problem which surgery can usually solve. Another possibility is an hormonal disorder diagnosed by a ready response to clomophene (Clomid) which acts on the pituitary gland. Occasional spontaneous cycles do occur, and are then normal and fertile. Other secondary causes (i.e. triggered by some other illness or condition) can be due to failure of the reproductive organs, a closed hymen, chromosomal abnormalities, ovarian cysts or anorexia.

PRECOCIOUS PUBERTY

This is breast development starting at or before the age of seven. (According to the *Guiness Book of Records*, pregnancy has been recorded in a five year old.) It usually represents one extreme of normal although, rarely, a hormone-secreting tumour may be responsible. The main problems are stunted growth, due to premature fusion of the growing ends of the bones; an early, inappropriate sexual desire; and aggressive behavioural problems.

EARLY MENARCHE

This means starting to menstruate before the age of ten. Sometimes, no explanation can be found (I started a month before my tenth birthday and there was nothing wrong). Medical causes include benign (non-cancerous) ovarian tumours, and early hormone release due to factors such as meningitis or encephalitis, which is brain inflammation.

PROBLEMS OF THE FIRST YEAR

Menstruation for the first year or so is often irregular, with blood loss varying between scanty to heavy, and the discomfort from absent or mild to severe. In fact, often ovulation does not start until the second year. While the sex hormones are sufficiently active to cause a reaction in the womb lining so bleeding occurs, it is insufficient to trigger ovulation. Around 90% of girls in the UK do know about periods in advance, but the arrival of the ‚menarche when no information has been given beforehand, can be highly traumatic.

A recent (1992/3) survey carried out by a Dr. S Prendergast on behalf of the Cambridge Health Promotion Research Trust, showed that the menarche came as a frightening shock for one in ten girls. Much misery and physical discomfort can be avoided by the giving of simple information on this entirely normal aspect of life – an open approach to the whole topic of periods and what they signify – well before they are expected to start.

PROBLEMS AT SCHOOL

The Prendergast survey also revealed the lack of toilet facilities in schools: more than 70% of the girls interviewed, described these as inadequate; in some instances, cloakrooms and toilets were locked during lessons, and the problem was especially acute for the 10% of girls who started menstruation at primary school.

Schoolgirls, generally, worried about obtaining access to sanitary protection at school while avoiding the notice and intrusion of boys. School authorities could help by adopting sympathetic policies over both cloakroom and toilet access and personal secure lockers; and by stocking sanitary towels and tampons. Other worries, linked to period pain, centred on its effects on performance in examinations and competitive sports; none, though, had been offered a combined oral contraceptive (see below).

WHAT YOU SHOULD DO

• Ask parents, sisters, aunts etc., or an older friend or teacher about periods if no-one's mentioned them to you;

• AND get a book out of the library – the most detailed, well-intended verbal advice is often inaccurate!

• Keep a couple of aspirin or paracetamol on you to deal with tummy cramps (avoid aspirin if you are under 12). Natural remedies also help, as you'll see later.

• Let someone know if facilities are poor or lacking; your friends will be suffering, too. If you're too embarrassed, write a note to your class teacher.

CHOICE OF SANITARY PROTECTION

Tampons are a popular choice of sanitary protection because they avoid the odour problem, allow you to wear the shortest of garments, swimwear, sportswear etc. without producing that horrible, telltale bulge, and are perfectly adequate provided you choose the correct size for your needs and remember to change them regularly (otherwise embarrassing overflow can occur).

They may need the backup protection of a sanitary towel if your periods are heavy (see Chapter 3). Modern towels stick on to the inside of your panties, covering the gusset – thicker, absorbent bit in the area of the crotch. You can buy towels and tampons from supermarkets, grocers' shops, chemists, drug stores, coin machines in Ladies' Cloakrooms. Individually-wrapped towels and tampons fit easily into your pocket, handbag or a biggish purse. Tampons normally flush away down the loo; some towels are supposed to disappear in this way, too; maybe they do, when anyone else tries, but you can depend on it that, if you're already having a bad day, *yours* will be the horror that remains oozing bloodily around the lavatory pan, refusing to acknowledge its biodegradable nature and eventually blocking the outlet pipe.

If you're in a hotel or public loo, at least you can hopefully remain anonymous; it's a different story at home or in someone else's bathroom. It's easier to shove used towels in bins or incinerators provided; or, if they're not in evidence, wrap the thing up in masses of toilet tissue and hide it in the bottom of your handbag. Just don't forget it's there, and pull it out hours later.

If you have just started your periods and/or haven't experienced full penetrative sex, you may experience difficulty in inserting even the most slimline tampon. Use towels for the time being, and experiment when you are alone and have plenty of time. It helps to grease the tampon tip with Vaseline, and take a deep breath then exhale before inserting it in the entrance to your vagina.

Technically, tampons rupture the hymen and destroy virginity, but this is not at all the same thing as losing your virginity through intercourse. Some girls have practically no hymen anyway, either because they were born that way or because 'stretchy' sports like hurdling, long and high jump, riding, have gradually worn the hymen membrane away.

Three further words of advice to tampon users: (1) Toxic shock syndrome is a form of septicaemia (blood poisoning) that affects a small number of women yearly. It is caused by bacterial toxins entering the bloodstream, from harmful bugs allowed to develop in blood-soaked tampons left in place for hours on end – a perfect breeding medium for them.

Symptoms can include fever, nausea, loss of appetite and faintness, stomach pains and, unless treated, sudden profound fall in blood pressure (clinical shock), which can be fatal in the absence of expert medical treatment.

(2) Other vaginal and cervical infections can result from tampon abuse. Avoid tampons if you have any of the symptoms, such as a coloured, offensive discharge, severe soreness or irritation.

(3) If you 'lose' a tampon inside, don't panic. If you relax into a squatting position, you may be able to hook it down with a (clean) index finger. It helps to empty your bladder and bowels first, then 'bear down' as though you were straining to pass urine; this helps to bring the end of the tampon down within reach. If you're unsuccessful, GPs and Casualty doctors are adepts – this is a fairly frequent dilemma.

CHANGES ENCOUNTERED FROM MENARCHE TO MENOPAUSE

Between the ages of 25 and 35, women are least likely to seek specialist gynaecological advice about serious problems (but most likely to seek medical advice for menstrual difficulties). The 20s and 30s are also prime time for having babies. At a time when new 'diseases' are discovered weekly (often promoted by the adornment of syndrome) something called The Shift or the Other 'Change' has recently come into vogue (Adele Cherreson,

1993). This refers to subtle changes in appearance, menstrual cycle and sex drive that herald the menopause from the late 20s onwards! Ms Cherreson advises us to watch out for fine hairs on the face, thighs and toes (!), skin-tone changes and crow's feet, love handles, a thickening waistline, cyclical problems including PMS, as 'decade by decade our systems adjust to ageing'.

Personally I would not dream of advising young, healthy women to start watching out for signs of decline and decay. Cherreson quotes gynaecologist Dr. Jean Ginsburg, who feels that 'healthy pre-planning can achieve a feeling of well being around the time of the menopause'. She says: 'In the same way that women nowadays go into training (sic) for pregnancy, they should maintain a certain level of health if they want a problem-free menopause'.

How likely would you be to eat, exercise and relax sensibly before you're 40 because you wanted to minimise possible future hot flushes (not everyone suffers from them, anyway)? As Miss Ginsburg recommends, i.e. quit smoking, stay active, take dietary calcium and don't drown yourself in alcohol ('there's nothing wrong with a glass of wine a day'!), but for goodness sake do so in order to extract maximum pleasure and satisfaction here and now; an easier menopause may well be a bonus.

Don't start quizzing your appearance and menstrual pattern for age-related changes for up to 30 years before they really get going!

It's true that fertility peaks in our 20s and early 30s (but look at the number of women starting families well into their 40s or later). PMS (see Chapter 7) also tends to worsen as the menopause approaches, but its main natural remedy takes this into account. Metabolism inevitably falls if we exercise less, but middle-age spread is *not* inevitable – expecting it means accepting it and Bob's your uncle, you've got it!

In the next chapter we'll look at heavy and irregular bleeding which affects all age groups and can be distressing until you understand causes and cures.

Chapter Three

HEAVY PERIODS

The ancient Greeks had a word for heavy periods or, rather, two words (men – month, and rhegynai – to burst forth) which have given rise to our modern medical term 'menorrhagia'. Sufferers of severe forms of this condition will agree it is apt: heavy flooding of menstrual blood can resemble a river or dam bursting its banks to swamp everything in the immediate vicinity.

Menorrhagia is a common complaint: 31 out of every 1000 women per doctor's panel seek medical advice about it every year; GPs have a 4% chance of seeing a case whenever they are consulted by a woman of reproductive years; and *you* have a 10–15% chance of being one of them. Despite this, identifying some of the less dramatic degrees of menorrhagia can be difficult. As with the question 'how long is a piece of string?', the problem of 'how heavy is heavy?' remains unanswerable; it amounts, essentially, to what you are used to.

WHEN IS HEAVY, HEAVY?

A persistent increase in personal monthly flow is the most usual stimulus to a visit to the surgery, yet doctors continue, irritatingly, to define menorrhagia as a menstrual blood loss in excess of 80 mls. Actual volume of blood passed per vagina is hard to measure and, in practice, patients do (or should) get taken seriously when they describe losing significantly more blood than is usual for them. Graphic accounts are also common of clots or 'bits' in the blood, and suddenly needing extra sanitary protection, often in the form of sanitary towels.

Both these symptoms can be distressing for someone accustomed to a 'normal' flow, who has used tampons for years and who has shunned pads as unattractive memorabilia of an earlier, darker Age. However, we vary enormously as individuals with respect to the amount of protection we think we need. A gynaecologist writing in a 1988 issue of the Journal of Sexual Medicine, for instance, mentioned that one woman used fifteen sanitary pads to collect 35 mls. of blood, while another used the same number and brand to collect 1500 mls.

Sanitary protection has, in fact, become a major business. The UK market, valued at £200 million in 1991, employs more than 12,000 people, and the average woman spends in excess of £17 annually on its products.

Severe menorrhagia, which can be incapacitating, can interfere with a person's lifestyle as surely as urinary incontinence. Sports become impossible, and work, social activities, even a quick whip round the supermarket suddenly have to be planned around the accessibility of local loos. Some sufferers have to plug the flow with the largest available tampons, and protect themselves further with babies' nappies or adult incontinence pads. Physical comfort, self-confidence and self-esteem, not to mention libido, can all be affected.

Clinically it is diagnosed when monthly blood-loss exceeds 80 mls. Another downside of defining heavy menstruation so precisely, is that around 60% of women complaining of it technically do not suffer from it!

Bleeding is often heavier after stopping oral contraceptives; but this may be no more than a return to normal (the average menstrual loss is about 55 mls.) compared to the reduced flow while on the Pill. In more than half of the women with menorrhagia, no underlying disorder can be found.

CAUSES

1. COMMON POSSIBILITIES

Some experts believe that abnormal levels of prostaglandin (hormone-like chemicals – see

Chapter 4 on Painful Periods) may be responsible. Other possibilities include endocrine imbalance e.g. an underactive thyroid gland, failure to ovulate; blood-clotting problems – e.g. carrying the haemophilia gene, poorly-controlled anticoagulant treatment; IUCDs (intrauterine contraceptive devices, the Coil); and local disorders affecting the womb or pelvis. The last mentioned group is by far the most usual cause.

2. FIBROIDS AND OTHER BENIGN TUMOURS

These non-cancerous tumours of the womb can be largely external, growing into the abdominal cavity from the outer surface of the womb to which they are attached only by a stalk; or within the wall tissue itself; or just beneath the mucous layer that covers the endometrial lining. Where they develop determines the symptoms, and fibroids at the last two sites typically cause painless menorrhagia by enlarging or distorting the uterine cavity.

The growth of fibroids is clearly influenced by ovarian hormones because they develop during the reproductive years, especially during pregnancy, when they can outgrow their blood supply and wither, causing internal bleeding. They are commoner in black women, and their growth is enhanced by late first pregnancy (i.e. after the age of 30). They regress after the menopause, usually becoming impregnated with glassy material called hyaline. Probably arising from vascular tissue, fibroids vary in size from a grape to a football, and several are usually present at the same time. 'Submucous' fibroids growing by stalks from the womb lining may be partly expelled through the cervix where they can get strangulated, causing severe bleeding.

This type of fibroid can also be mistaken for a polyp – a flattish or stalked growth of the endometrium sometimes containing a bit of fibrous or muscular tissue from the womb wall. Usually, although not always, benign, endometrial polyps measure between one and five cms. across, and can give rise to severe irregular vaginal bleeding, as well as heavy bleeding.

Other benign conditions of the womb associated with heavy periods include (giving their medical names): adenomyoma – enlargement of the uterus in response to endometriosis (see below) which also causes pain; and uterine hypertrophy, in which the size of the womb may increase two or threefold, usually during the last decade of reproductive life as a result of hormonal changes.

3. ENDOMETRIOSIS
A common cause of heavy periods, endometriosis is a condition in which endometrial tissue is found elsewhere than the lining of the womb, such as

the ovaries, wall of the bladder or rectum, the vagina, ligaments supporting the womb or Fallopian tubes, crevices in the pelvis between major organs, and scars of the abdominal wall or uterus. Deposits have also been found elsewhere in the body, e.g. the lungs, causing a blood-stained cough especially troublesome during menstruation, and also small, vascular tumours of the arms and legs; but both are rareties.

Theories about how endometrial cells get displaced to these sites, abound. There is evidence to suggest that retrograde menstruation may be responsible – in which womb lining cells travel up the Fallopian tubes during a period, and out into the pelvic or abdominal cavity. They may also migrate along the veins or lymph vessels draining the womb; or develop from tissues such as the lining of the abdominal or pelvic cavities derived from common embryonic stock.

The symptoms of endometriosis arise largely because the errant cells respond to oestrogen just like ordinary endometrial tissue, and are unrelated to the extent of the disease – widespread deposits may be discovered during an internal examination carried out for some other reason where they can be detected as hard, tender nodules, or as tender masses in the ovaries, never having given a clue to their existence; while small clumps can produce marked effects. Infertility may be the only sign:

but menorrhagia is common, as are pain on deep intercourse and period cramps. If the ovaries are affected, the cycles may alter, usually becoming shorter; and blood may appear cyclically in the urine if deposits are found in the bladder wall or kidney tubes (ureters), although it may well pass unnoticed.

Endometriosis can affect teenagers, but is commoner in women in their thirties and forties, especially Caucasians in developed countries. There are probable links with being sterilized and with a low number of (or absence of) pregnancies. The deposits regress during pregnancy under the influence of progesterone, and again after the menopause when oestrogen levels drop.

4. PELVIC INFLAMMATORY DISEASE

This is a broad term covering infection of the tubes, ovaries, tissue connecting the genital organs, and other pelvic tissues such as the wall of the large bowel or the bladder, usually as a result of adhesions. Its chief features are lower abdominal pain and painful intercourse; but it also commonly causes menorrhagia (and/or irregular vaginal bleeding); increased (often offensive) vaginal discharge; period pains; bladder symptoms such as frequency, scalding etc.; pain in the rectum (proclitis); fever, nausea and vomiting.

Pelvic inflammatory disease is, in fact, a total pain from everyone's point of view, doctors and patients alike. Like cystitis, it can recur time and again for no apparent reason, clearing up briefly after treatment and rearing its ugly head again just when its victim is starting to forget her GP's surgery appointments number. Even with the most carefully performed tests and scrupulously detailed history, PID is identified accurately in no more than 66% of cases. As tutors in gynaecology are forever pointing out to medical students, the acronym stands as validly for Poorly Identified Diagnosis as it does for the illness itself.

Part of the problem is the wide spectrum of symptoms, giving ground for highly individual profiles in sufferers. Symptoms are, in fact, so often unreliable that many specialists now look for three or more in addition to lower pelvic pain and painful penetration, before considering using the PID label. Established predisposing factors such as an intrauterine contraceptive device (IUCD) or sexually transmitted diseases in the patient and/or her partner, are useful pointers. Even true recurrences of PID have to be carefully differentiated from the periodic bouts of chronic lower abdominal pain in the absence of infection, that continue to harass around 20% of women after they've officially recovered.

Other possible causes of PID include tissue damage, possibly following a termination or delivery, usually with bacteria from the gut or vagina; blood-borne organisms e.g. in a patient with tuberculosis; and infection from other abdominal organs such as a ruptured abscess of the appendix or of the large bowel, in a woman with diverticulitis (inflammation of tiny, finger-like projections of gut lining that rupture outwards, under pressure, through the large bowel's muscular walls).

In case you suffer from it, it's worth noting that there are two main forms of pelvic inflammatory disease:

(1) the acute sort, which is not really connected with menorrhagia, figuring inflamed, infected Fallopian tubes (salpingitis) from which pus escapes and infects other pelvic areas and organs and

(2) chronic PID, which can develop after an attack of the acute variety if treatment is inadequate or delayed; adhesions usually form between the Fallopian tubes, ovaries and other structures, the natural folds of the membrane lining the tubes, together with the hair-like cilia (see page 7) are destroyed, and the uterus gets anchored down tightly into an abnormal retroverted position, (leaning backwards instead of forwards relative to the cervix).

CONSULTING A DOCTOR

Information your doctor will want if you consult him/her about heavy periods, includes: how long you have suffered from the problem; was the change from your usual menstrual loss, gradual or sudden; how long your periods last and how often they arrive; plus details of contraceptive methods (if any), and medication.

A physical examination ought to and probably will, otherwise make sure that it does, include both a general check (breasts, tummy, blood pressure) and an 'internal'. This involves the doctor feeling the pelvic organs to assess their shape and size, and identify any tender areas (e.g. in endometriosis, or pelvic inflammatory disease), with one finger in the vagina and the other hand pressing gently on the abdominal wall. The next stage is inspecting the cervix and its lower opening (called the os), via a speculum to check for a protruding polyp or fibroid, or a cervical erosion (see Chapter 5). Next would come a cervical smear, and a high vaginal swab for bacteriological examination should signs of infection e.g. offensive discharge, be present.

A routine blood count should also be performed: a low haemoglobin level suggests iron deficiency anaemia, high numbers of white cells suggest infection. Other possibilities, depending on findings and individual case history, are: tests of the blood-clotting mechanism; and of thyroid function: menorrhagia is occasionally triggered by hypothyroidism (underactive thyroid).

Further tests can be carried out in hospital. A common example is sampling (biopsy) of the womb lining using the suction method in the out-patient department without anaesthesia (but, per-haps, sedation), or a standard D & C (dilation and curettage – womb scrape) on an inpatient basis under anaesthesia.

This is mandatory for women over forty with heavy menstrual bleeding to eliminate womb cancer; but could be safely deferred in younger women unless their bleeding was severe, they also had intermenstrual bleeding, and/or hormone treatment was either contraindicated or unsuc-cessful. Some specialised centres are able to offer hysteroscopy (direct inspection of the uterine lining), excellent for revealing endometrial polyps (see Chaper 6) or fibroids passed over during a D & C.

TREATMENT

Treatment for menorrhagia can be medical or surgical, and obviously depends on the cause, but should also take into account, wherever possible, the patient's wishes: e.g. wanting to start/add to a family, in which case a medical approach (rather than surgery) should be adopted when there is no pelvic or other abnormality dictating otherwise. Obligatory surgery for, perhaps, endometriotic nodules or large or multiple fibroids, should – the current, patient-orientated view is said to go – be carried out as conservatively as possible in women who want to remain fertile. (And most women do, even those who have no intention of becoming pregnant.)

1. MEDICAL

Drugs can reduce menstrual blood loss by enhancing blood clotability; or inhibiting (possibly aggravating) natural hormone prostaglandins (e.g. mefanamic acid, Ponstan). Progestogens e.g. norethisterone in the second half of the cycle, and oral contraceptives in women under 30 who also happen to want contraceptive protection, also work well. Some doctors prescribe the fertility drug clomiphene (Clomid) for women with menorrhagia linked with failure to ovulate; many sufferers claim to have found relief but there is little objective evidence to show that it really reduces heavy menstrual bleeding, and it is probably best confined to women who actually want to become pregnant.

Danazol (Danol) is also often used successfully for menorrhagia, and should be taken daily, without a break, for however long proves necessary. It is widely prescribed for patients with endometriosis, but recent studies have shown that the better-tolerated goserelin (Zoladex), given by subcutaneous injection every 28 days, is equally effective

45

in controlling pain by up to 50% (and relieving other symptoms). Goserelin tended to cause menopausal-like symptoms such as hot flushes and sweats, and vaginal dryness; but danazol produced androgenic side effects e.g. increased body and facial hair.

Medical treatment for pelvic inflammatory disease usually consists of one or more antibiotics. Only certain pathogens (disease-causing organisms) are sufficiently virulent to overcome the natural, protective barrier provided structurally and chemically by the cervix and its mucus. (Neisseria) gonorrhoea and Chlamydia (trachomatis) causing genital infections of the same names, are both common culprits. Secondary infection extending further into the pelvis then usually develops, or can arise from other causes such as an IUCD (see above) which increases the risks of pelvic inflammatory disease by up to ten times.

Specimens for bacteriological investigation can be taken from the cervical canal, urethra, vagina; or from the ends of the Fallopian tubes and pelvic pockets during a laparoscopy (view of inside of abdomen by inserting a lighted tube through the tummy wall) or laparotomy (opening up the abdominal wall to inspect organs first-hand). Recent research has also shown that a biopsy of the endometrium can be a sensitive and specific diagnostic technique. Contact tracing is vital when findings are positive: treatment is normally started as soon as the diagnosis is reached. If there's reason to suspect a sexually-transmitted disease (or one is actually identified), usual drugs would be tetracycline or erythromycin for Chlamydia, and a penicillin or spectinomycin for gonorrhoea.

2. SURGICAL
This has already been mentioned in connection with polyps, fibroids and endometriosis. Womb polyps and fibroids can sometimes be removed at specialised centres with the aid of hysteroscopy (see above): otherwise, hysterectomy is offered to both older women and to the increasing numbers of younger women who have completed their families and are reluctant to take drugs indefinitely.

3. NATURAL REMEDIES
Herbal: when linked to congestion of the pelvic blood vessels (and therefore congestive period pains), life root, shepherd's purse and white dead nettle are indicated. When anaemia is present and fragile capillaries that make you bleed or bruise readily) – ladies' mantle, black haw, beth root may be useful.

Homoeopathic remedies – Arsenicum, Chamomile.

Aromatherapy – Heavy bleeding may respond very well to cypress, geranium or rose.

Dietary supplement: Iron deficiency anaemia – around 10% of women are believed to suffer from this in Britain; the Committee on Medical Aspects of Food Policy (COMA), DoH, 1991) found that the Recommended National Intake (similar to the RDA) for iron is enough (18 mg daily) to cover the needs of 90% of women, leaving about 10% with higher menstrual losses and higher dietary iron needs. The panel concluded that for these women, additional iron is best taken as iron supplements; and dietary supplementation may be needed by mothers with low iron stores.

My personal choice of iron supplement is Feroglobin B12; it comes as a liquid or sustained release capsules, and when I first sampled it at a health exhibition three years ago, I loved its malt, orange and honey flavour. One teaspoon (5 ml) or one capsule of Feroglobin B12 supplies 10 mg of iron, and other vital nutrients needed for the absorption and utilisation of iron by the body. These include 8 B vitamins including the elusive B12; folic acid; trace elements zinc, copper and manganese; and the essential amino acid lysine. Feroglobin comes from Vitabiotics. It costs £3.95 for 200 mls liquid, or £4.95 for 30 capsules, from chemists and health stores.

Chapter Four

PAINFUL PERIODS

Period pain, known medically as dysmenorrhoea, is a common problem affecting all women to some degree during their reproductive years. A UK survey during the 80s showed that 6.8 million (58.6%) of the 11.6 million women aged fifteen to forty-four who took part, experienced sufficient discomfort to require some sort of remedy, either self-administered or prescribed: and that more than half of them suffered pain every time they menstruated, 2.6 million rating their pain as severe.

SYMPTOMS

Period pain is most often felt in the lower abdomen – the region known as supra-pubic because it is located immediately above the pubic bone that forms the front of the pelvis, just below where you can feel your bladder when it is full. It is a deep, penetrating pain often extending into the back and down the inside of the thighs and around the genitals. The spasms and cramps come in bouts, starting up, reaching a peak and then dying away, and a brief lull can easily persuade you – wrongly – that it has finally disappeared. Caused by muscular contractions of the womb's walls, the discomfort can be both severe and hard to pin to an exact spot. Period pain cannot, therefore, be reached like a bruise or strain for the purpose of rubbing better; although massage of the lower tummy and back can help if carried out correctly, preferably using an appropriate aromatherapy essence.

Other symptoms you may experience in addition to cramps, include headache, dizziness, nausea and vomiting, lethargy, exhaustion and depression, irritability and poor concentration, fainting attacks and either constipation or diarrhoea. Most women tolerate the discomfort, requiring, at most, just an occasional pain-killer or anti-nauseant; yet a few, usually in their teens and twenties, experience all or nearly all of these symptoms and, for them, dysmenorrhoea represents a serious disruption to their social, domestic and working lives either in employment or at school or college, as well as to personal relationships and peace of mind.

Various theories have been put forward to account for this important condition; it's interesting to look at them since they help to explain how and why certain treatments and self-help methods work.

PRIMARY DYSMENORRHOEA

The commonest type of dysmenorrhoea starts a year or so after the menarche (first period), and either comes on a few hours before, or coincides with the start of, bleeding. The pelvic and back pain, though they can be severe, are normally over within twenty-four hours and often respond well to simple remedies.

1. CAUSES

Known as primary because it is not triggered by some other illness or gynaecological condition, this dysmenorrhoea is associated with ovulation (which is why it is usually absent during the first year of menstruation before ovulation gets under way, see Chapter 1). The muscular spasms that cause the pain are believed to occur in response to increased amounts of a prostaglandin, F 2a, from the walls of the uterus, present in the menstrual blood. Other symptoms such as headache, nausea, faintness are due to the effects of this prostaglandin on other organs which it reaches via the bloodstream. Diarrhoea can become troublesome when the autonomic nervous system controlling digestion and bowel movements, is disturbed.

(Prostaglandins are dealt with in more detail in Chapter 7.)

2. OTHER ISSUES

Psychological factors can also play a part in primary dysmenorrhoea: surveys have shown that women with period cramps who either fail to discuss menstruation with their daughters, or talk negatively about it (in terms of suffering, being unwell, the 'curse' etc.), tend to have dysmenorrhoeic daughters.

3. WILL IT GET ANY BETTER?

Unlike PMS which worsens with age, primary dysmenorrhoea becomes less severe from around the mid-twenties onwards, especially after the birth of the first baby – possibly because the cervix is so widely stretched during delivery that subsequent stretching during periods to allow the escape of menstrual flood (part of the source of the pain), is no longer an issue. Primary dysmenorrhoea is also known as spasmodic, to differentiate it from the other form of the complaint (congestive dysmenorrhoea).

SECONDARY DYSMENORRHOEA

Here the sufferer is almost invariably an older woman whose periods have in the past been relatively trouble free. It occurs as a result of some identifiable reason such as an IUCD (intrauterine contraceptive device, the Coil), or a disorder like those discussed in this book, e.g. endometriosis, pelvic inflammatory disease, fibroids.

Secondary dysmenorrhoea is 'congestive' rather than 'spasmodic', because the pain-producing mechanism lies in the small blood vessels (capillaries) and veins of the pelvis and womb, which dilate and become over-suffused with blood for a time just before period blood loss starts. The pain is, therefore, typically felt in the day(s) approaching menstruation towards and at the end of the cycle, and gets worse as the next period approaches; although there is doubtless a congestive element in the ordinary, spasmodic variety.

Congestive period pain is also more constant, i.e. stays on a plateau rather than rising and falling in peaks and troughs; and it is more often felt deep in the pelvis and lower back, than in the central or lower tummy. If untreated, it tends to worsen with age. The emotions often play a part, perhaps originating in distress over menstruation during the teen years. This element is especially likely to be present in cases of 'pelvic congestion syndrome' (see below), which this sort of period pain gets mislabelled as, when no underlying cause is found (this happens in at least 50% of cases).

CONSULTING A DOCTOR

When pelvic pain – or any pain – is very severe, there is no real problem about whether or not to consult a doctor; the question simply resolves itself into: 'How soon can I get there?' Moderate, niggling, intermittent pain is far harder to decide about.

We vary a lot in how much pain we can bear, and for how long. Factors such as prolonged physical or mental stress, emotional trauma, illness and convalescence, poor diet, inadequate sleep, age, sex, general health and our surroundings can all undermine our stoicism and resilience. Only you can decide when pain you are experiencing requires professional help. The general consensus is that if dysmenorrhoea is disrupting your life; keeping you away from work, school or social occasions, even proving a recurrent irritation or embarrassment, then you should seek medical advice.

TREATMENT

1. MEDICAL

Most of the pain of dysmenorrhoea, as opposed to the other symptoms, responds well to soluble aspirin (take paracetamol instead if you are under twelve, suffer from peptic ulcers or gastritis, are on a permanent course of anticoagulants, e.g.

Warfarin, or cannot take aspirin for any other reason). Aspirin is the simplest, longest established and most familiar of a group of drugs known as NSAIDs (non-steroidal anti-inflammatory drugs). Other examples are mefenamic acid (Ponstan), ibuprofen (Brufen, Codafen) and piroxicam (Feldene), all of which are also prescribed for rheumatoid arthritis, in which inflammatory prostaglandins play a part in causing pain.

Doctors often treat dysmenorrhoea with NSAIDs, which work by suppressing the pain-triggering prostaglandins. In theory, they ought to have some effect on non-pelvic symptoms; but other, preferably simple, medicines are often required, at least at first. Examples are prochlorperazine (Stemetil) for nausea and dizzy spells, diphenoxylate hydrochloride (Lomotil) or loperamide (Immodium), which you can buy for diarrhoea, and ispaghula husks (Fybogel) for constipation. Hyoscine (Buscopan) and alverine (Spasmonal) are two anti-spasmodics that act directly on the womb wall, where they relieve painful muscular cramps.

After analgesics, antispasmodics and prostaglandin inhibitors, the combined oral contraceptive pill is the mainstay of treatment, because it suppresses ovulation with which dysmenorrhoea is closely linked. Familiar instances are Loostrin, Microgynon and Eugynon, all combining various doses of oestrogen and progestogen. Progestogens such as norothisterone (Utovlan, Menzol) or dydrogesterone (Duphastson) are useful for relieving period cramps when contraception is not required. They are normally taken from day five to day 26 of the cycle.

2. NATURAL REMEDIES

Herbal – cramp bark, black haw, blue cohosh. For painful cramps, Agnus castus works well.

For *ovulatory pain*, and for *congestive dysmenorrhoea* and other symptoms caused by pelvic inflammatory disease (PID) – helonias root with Echinacea, combined with beth root, blue cohosh or wild indigo as required.

Homoeopathic remedies – Mag. phos. (Magnesium phosphate) Gelsemium (especially for painful periods if and when they start after the menarche). Chamomile or Viburnum for pelvic cramps and backache; Aloe or Nit. Ac. (nitric acid) for a 'bearing down' sort of pain.

FAILURE TO RESPOND – THE LAST RESORT

Period pains that fail to respond to the above measures, need further investigations. Referral to a consultant gynaecologist would normally be the next stage, and while he/she might then offer you a D & C (dilation and curettage, 'womb scrape') to see whether stretching the opening of the cervix may help (see above), this is now considered outdated and ultrasound or a laparoscopy would be a more likely choice.

Either of these techniques would stand a good chance of revealing other causes of dysmenorrhoea such as those linked with the secondary kind, i.e. endometriosis, fibroids. This can make sense in young women with intractable (primary) period pain because, although most dysmenorrhoea at that age is associated with ovulation, other explanations usually confined to older age groups cannot be ruled out without tests. Treatment for these complaints is as we have seen elsewhere in this book: i.e. removal of fibroids if fertility is an issue (or of the womb if it is not); medical treatment or surgery for deposits of endometriosis; bacteriological investigations and courses of the appropriate antibiotics for pelvic inflammatory disease (PID).

PELVIC CONGESTION SYNDROME (PCS)

This is a hotch potch of pelvic and PMS-like symptoms, usually diagnosed only by default when other disorders have been eliminated. It is generally said to have a 'psychosomatic origin', it probably has; but, like other emotionally generated complaints, this makes it no easier to bear. One way of telling, is that pain due to a diseased pelvic organ, may well wake you during the night; pain (or any other symptom) resulting from psychological causes very rarely does this.

Women of any age can be affected, but PCS is commoner after 30. Dysmenorrhoea is usually the main symptom, followed by deep dyspareunia (pain on penetrative sex), a non-offensive vaginal discharge, and bloating with weight gain due to fluid retention. Unsurprisingly, most sufferers lose interest in sex, at least temporarily, and are unable to reach climax. Physical discomfort and pain often combine with the sexual aspect of this syndrome to turn a diagnosable and treatable, if complex, complaint into a disruptive menace detrimental to self esteem, personal partnerships and well being.

The most important alternatives that need to be ruled out – by laparoscopy – before identifying pelvic congestive syndrome, are endometriosis and pelvic inflammatory disease. Few women with pelvic pain enjoy being 'mauled about' as abdominal, pelvic and 'internal' examinations are often described; and those with PCS can be very difficult to examine because, intercourse suddenly having become painful, they find it impossible to relax. The entire pelvis usually feels tender, and the womb, mottled, bulky and flexed back on its own axis out of its normal, forward position, i.e., 'retroverted'. There is no underlying disease of the womb itself; but a hysterectomy may be suggested for a woman whose family is complete and evidence found of thickened, fibrosed uterine support ligaments, and congested and swollen veins.

IF YOU CONTINUE TO SUFFER

Some women continue to experience pelvic pain even after their womb, ovaries and tubes have been removed. Experts urge that psychologically pain-dependent patients should be identified as early in the proceedings as possible, to save them from needless pelvic investigations and, possibly, surgery. Sometimes, a laparoscopy producing a sound bill of health, relieves PCS symptoms in highly anxious patients.

Psychosexual counselling combined with contraceptive advice and general health care, is often successful when pain and sexual relationship problems are particular issues. Because of the emotional element in this condition, many patients also respond well to alternative treatment methods such as acupuncture, or homoeopathic or herbal remedies prescribed by qualified practitioners.

Chapter Five

IRREGULAR/MISSED PERIODS

Periods work according to the unique rhythmicity and timescale of our biological clock and, under certain conditions, are just as likely as more tangible timepieces to slow down, accelerate or stop.

To appreciate how various factors can upset our fine tuning, it's important to remember (Chapter 1) the biochemical subservience of the pituitary gland (which regulates the menstrual cycle), to the hypothalamus – the comprehensive control HQ in the midbrain – and, via the hypothalamus, to the 'higher centres' of grey matter that concentrate and store our thoughts and emotions.

Unsurpisingly, physical and emotional highs and lows, shock, worry, stress, diet, medication, lifestyle changes, severe fatigue, illness and drugs all effect menstruation, and must be considered before other causes for irregularity or amenorrhoea (absence of periods), with which, of course, they can also coincide. We'll deal with them first in the *Causes* section.

Irregular periods are a major nuisance: it is inconvenient and, of course, worrying not to know when you will next bleed, for how long, or what sort of gap to expect between subsequent periods. It is important to find out, if possible, whether your cycle itself is upset, whether you are having regular periods interspersed with intermenstrual bleeding, or irregular bleeding unassociated with menstruation. The cause, and the source of non-period blood loss, then has to be traced to the uterus, genitals or elsewhere.

POSSIBLE CAUSES

Here is a passage from an article by Dr. Carn-Bains, a GP in Guildford, Surrey, which appeared in a January 1993 issue of a doctors' weekly newspaper under the title of: *Through the minefield of menstrual malady*: 'Scanty, prolonged or irregular periods are unlikely to be more than a normal physiological variation. Irregular periods caused by anovulatory cycles are quite common at the extremes of reproductive life. The temptation to force regularity on the pubertal girl by giving the oral contraceptive Pill should be avoided unless contraception is truly needed.

'Intermenstrual and post-coital bleeding should always be taken seriously. Both may be caused by uterine and vaginal pathologies detectable on examination. Erosions, cervical polyps, endometrial and cervical carcinomas are possible causes. Unexplained bleeding of this variety should be referred for a second opinion, especially in older women. Postmenopausal bleeding without HRT (hormone replacement therapy) should produce a high index of suspicion of endometrial carcinoma, especially if more than a year has elapsed since the cessation of periods.

'Many women now seek help from alternative medicine and as long as the bleeding is only dysfunctional and dysmenorrhoea (period pain) is not associated with pelvic pathology, there may be some benefit.'

CAUSES OF DYSFUNCTIONAL BLEEDING

The line between dysfunctional bleeding and a 'normal physiological variation', is blurred by subjective opinion and the idiosyncratic nature of the reproductive cycle. The difference is as much quantitative as qualitative, so here is a rule of thumb: relatively short intervals of stress, illness, change in personal environment or lifestyle can halt or destroy the regularity of normal periods – upsets that nine times out of ten, right themselves as soon as the stimulus disappears. Dysfunctional bleeding 'proper' is usually linked with an underlying hormonal problem, or graver physiological traumata such as sudden profound weight loss; serious overweight; and certain drugs.

1. HORMONES OUT OF LINE

Endocrine, i.e. glandular problems, can shift the length of the menstrual cycle or make it totally disordered and patternless, although in such cases particular care must be taken to eliminate the other most likely cause: some sort of local lesion of the womb, cervix or vagina. Endocrine disorders as such, can sometimes be proven by low or absent blood levels of progesterone. In practice, more knowledge on this subject is required (and being sought), and progesterone measurements would not be useful unless infertility is an associated problem. In fact, since irregular menses are commoner in the late and early reproductive years, women are more likely to require advice on contraception than enhancement of their fertility.

Usually with dysfunctional bleeding, the fourteen day interval mentioned elsewhere in this book, between ovulation and the next bleed, remains untouched, the time of ovulation itself becoming the variable factor. Occasionally, though, the second half of the menstrual cycle is atypically brief, because the corpus luteum (see page 9), which normally releases hormones to rebuild and thicken the womb lining after a period, fragments due to an inherent weakness about four days after ovulation.

2. SUDDEN LOSS OF WEIGHT

You can expect your periods to stop if your weight falls below 47kg (7 stone 4lbs) – official. But exceptions must of course be made for women of unusually petite frame. Rapid weight loss of 10% to 15% of your present weight can act as a metabolic 'red alert', warning of imminent starvation or similar biological crisis. The effect is that your fertility i.e. ability to ovulate goes on strike, and your periods cease until some sort of readjustment has been made.

Causes of prompt, profound weight loss include practically any factor that disrupts the appetite or cuts off food supply. Common examples are chronic pain, an accident, operation, convalescence, personal worries, anxiety illness, depression. Anorexia nervosa and bulimia, typically interfere with menstrual regularity and, if the anorectic spell persists, halt them altogether. These two eating disorders are traumatically difficult both to overcome and to treat: and the return of periods after weeks or months of amenorrhoea is a highly justified reason for jubilation for both the patient and her carer(s). (Boys and older men can become anorectic or bulimic, and share women's symptoms apart, of course, from any diminishment of their powers of reproduction.)

3. OBESITY

What a horrible word! And it's a condition linked with more anxiety, grief, aggression, loneliness and unhealthy lifestyle than most other common disorders put together. When really due to a 'glandular problem', e.g. thyroid, pituitary, ovarian, accompanying menstrual irregularity may also have a unique hormonal trigger and be difficult to diagnose and treat. But few cases of obesity are so caused. Nor are they usually due to 'heavy bones', fluid retention, heredity or food sensitivity.

A low metabolic rate (the slow burning of food fuel), too much food in relation to exercise, and/or appalling dietary habits that amount as much to an eating disorder as anorexia nervosa and bulimia – usually due to emotional or sexual deprivation and a consequent need for a substitute – are nearly always responsible. *However*, an overweight person often feels strongly motivated to claim otherwise.

Clinical obesity is a bodyweight more than 24% above that recommended for your height and build (which I haven't experienced but have certainly been heavy enough to know the anguish), is a result of the deposition of small quantities of oestrogen in the layers of surplus body fat. The more adipose tissue (body fat) you allow to collect, the more oestrogen is removed from the bloodstream for temporary storage, leaving too little for the efficient, regular maintenance of your menstrual cycle. This deficiency can and does have a negative influence on ovulation, producing irregular periods and/or amenorrhoea.

As with the other eating disorders, ovulation, regular menses and fertility practically always return when a woman's body weight is brought within normal limits.

4. DRUGS

Some medications can upset the menstrual cycle. Examples are treatment for thyroid or pituitary gland disorders; supplementary sex hormones as provided by the contraceptive Pill or HRT; antihypertensives for the treatment of high blood pressure; anti-anaemia drugs; tranquillisers; possibly some anti-depressants; anti-cancer treatments in the form of both cytotoxic drugs and radiotherapy. Quite apart from cancer treatment, malignant disease in itself can interfere with ovulation and menstrual regularity, even without involving the reproductive organs.

Consulting A Doctor

Although it is often impossible to tell what kind of bleeding you are experiencing, menstrual blood flow, even when irregular, can sometimes be identified by its pattern: an uninterrupted flow lasting for a few days, with most being passed within the first couple of days. Irregular periods are common and can usually be corrected; a diagnosis of dysfunctional bleeding is often indicated by the patient's history (e.g. significant weight loss due to crash dieting, or a long illness or period of severe anxiety), and is normally treated – after an examination to check the pelvic organs are healthy – with a combined oral contraceptive of oestrogen and progestogen.

TREATMENT

1. MEDICAL
When the bleeding is heavy, the choice of Pill will probably be one containing a relatively high dose of progestogen, such as Anovlar or Gynovlar, initially prescribed for only two to three cycles since many patients revert to their normal pattern when the medication is stopped. If oestrogen is unsuitable (see Chapter 9), then progestogen alone in the second half of the cycle, usually from days 15–25, works successfully in about 50% of cases by acting directly on the endometrium.

Certain progestogens such as danazol (Danol) and gestrinone (Dimetriose), often used for endometriosis, are sometimes chosen for their effect on the pituitary. In suppressing the release from this gland of the gonadotrophin hormones that control the ovaries, they work via a 'negative feedback' mechanism upon the pituitary which, in turn, reduces ovarian hormone production. Doses have to be tailored to a woman's particular needs, which means giving enough to correct the irregular bleeding, yet not enough to suppress the ovaries altogether and arrest menstruation. These progestogens also have to be taken throughout the month without interruption. Possible alternatives include drugs that modify the blood's clotting activity, and hysterectomy as a last resort.

2. NATURAL REMEDIES

Herbal remedies for irregular menstrual bleeding include: uterine stimulants such as blue cohosh, parsley, mugwort, rue or tonics like dong quai, helonias root, life root, motherwort.

Homoeopathic remedies – sepia, Senc (Senecium aureus, i.e. golden ragwort or squaw-weed).

Aromatherapy: to help bring on a period or increase scanty menstrual bleeding, try clary sage, myrrh or sage (which also ease cramps). Melissa can help regularise irregular periods.

Chapter Six

NON-MENSTRUAL BLEEDING

Irregular periods invariably have a benign (i.e. non-cancerous) cause, but non-menstrual bleeding is more often linked with some lesion or other on the cervix or in the womb (although there are other causes – see below), *and should be regarded as malignant until proven otherwise.* This will be a very frightening thing to read if you are merely browsing through this book hoping that it will shed light on bleeding that has bothered you for some time, but about which you haven't yet consulted your GP.

It is also the most important statement in this book. As a woman, you have a just under one in five (21%) chance of contracting cancer at some point in your life (men have a 23% chance). Excepting cancer of the breast, the commonest, which is not under discussion in this book, genital cancers taken together make up 18% of all female malignant growths. About 20% of the female population die from cancer, but the chances of surviving reproductive organ malignancy is relatively good compared with that of, say, the large bowel. The five year survival rate (percentage of women still living five years after diagnosis) is 70% with respect to cancer of the womb and up to 100% for pre-invasive cancer of the cervix (the earliest stage, that can be detected on routine cervical smear).

Genital tract cancer, generally, has a very good prognosis when detected and treated in the early stages; yet there's nothing wrong or shameful whatsoever, about procrastination or fear. There's everything wrong in the world with worrying privately about symptoms which you hope and pray will disappear; only to be driven, eventually, to seek help which, you then discover to your painful if transitory grief, and your family's protracted loss, has come too late.

THREE TYPES OF NON-MENSTRUAL BLEEDING

The three chief types of non-menstrual bleeding are referred to, purely descriptively, as intermenstrual (IMB), post-menopausal (PMB) and post-coital (PCB), which is bleeding after coitus or intercourse. Causes other than lesions (a lesion is a concentrated area of diseased tissue such as an ulcer or growth), include miscarriage (the commonest cause in young women), and breakthrough bleeding due to an oral contraceptive Pill

70

(especially the progestogen-only variety) that fails to inhibit bleeding from the endometrial womb lining. We are more concerned here with the lesions, though, for obvious reasons. The commonest include cervical erosion, polyp and cervical cancer; cancer of the endometrium; and cancers of the ovary and vulva.

BENIGN DISORDERS OF THE CERVIX

Millions of words are written yearly in the Western press about cervical disorders and their treatment. Cervical smears save thousands of lives yearly, but could save more if their importance, and simplicity, were more widely recognised. Nowadays, people generally, women especially, want to know the whys and wherefores of illnesses and tests before they take them seriously. So here is what happens to the cervix and, so far as it is possible to go in this book, how it happens.

The cervix or neck of the womb juts down for about an inch (2.5cm) into the upper part of the vagina where you can easily feel it with the tip of an index or middle finger. The lower opening of the cervical canal can be felt as a round, smooth-edged hollow or hole, through which menstrual blood leaves the body and sperm gain access to the uterus and Fallopian tubes.

The canal or endocervix is lined with column-shaped cells attached to an underlying membrane richly supplied with blood vessels, which gives it a translucent, bright crimson appearance. The columnar cells secrete mucus that varies in quantity and consistency at different phases of the menstrual cycle. The outer surface of the cervix (ectocervix) is covered, by way of contrast, with flat, plate-like hexagonal cells collectively called squamous epithelium, continuous with the membrane lining the rest of the vagina. Relatively smooth and thick, the underlying blood vessels do not shine through, so the ectocervix membrane is opaque and coloured a dullish pink. The line of demarcation between the two membranes is known (not particularly imaginatively, but entirely accurately) as the squamo-columnar junction.

These facts, far from being a mesmerisingly overdetailed and irrelevant space filler, are crucial to an understanding of both cervical erosions and cervical cancer, for it is in the region of this junction that cellular disorders most often occur, and from where smears should, therefore, be taken.

This important junction starts off in the pre-pubescent girl at or around the cervix's external os (opening), yet often ends up far removed from this region, somewhere on the outside of the ecto-cervix. In fact, during pregnancy, the endocervical membrane may cover most of the outside of the cervix. This seems to result from the relatively faster growth of the support tissues underlying the endocervix due to the influence of oestrogen, which carries the columnar lining membrane outwards with it.

(The junction may return to the external opening or even inside it after the menopause, as a result partly of tissue shrinkage, and partly of some of the columnar cells changing into squamous cells by a process called metaplasia.)

1. CERVICAL EROSION

The squamous cells of the ectocervix, geared chemically to the vaginal secretions, are frequently injured or destroyed by infection or childbirth or some other trauma. The more delicate columnar cells, used only to the more rarefied and protected environment within the cervical canal, creep down manfully to cover the damaged area, joining other columnar cells already brought there by the growth differential described above. Once in place, they succumb to attack by vaginal acidity and an unfamiliar bacteriological flora, they wither and die, and are continually replaced by more of their own kind. The process repeats itself, producing a red spot or 'erosion' of visible columnar cells at the edge of the cervical canal.

Cervical erosions may be symptomless, but often give rise to intermenstrual bleeding (IMB), post-coital bleeding (PCB) and/or a colourless or yellowy-brown, watery vaginal discharge. You may feel something slightly sore inside during intercourse. Erosions are commoner in women taking oral contraceptives, and after childbirth. They are not cancerous, nor do they predispose to cancer, but you need a smear to establish the health of the cervix as a whole. Erosions can safely be left alone if the smear is normal and they don't bleed, but bleeding erosions need to be treated. Cervical erosions can be frozen (without general anaesthesia) or cauterised (with a GA).

2. CERVICAL POLYP

This is a small, warty growth on a stalk, attached to, or protruding through the lower opening of, the cervix, and covered with lining or surface cells of either the squamous or the columnar type. Up to 10 mm in diameter, polyps are either spotted during a routine smear, or produce symptoms that lead to an internal examination and inspection of the cervix. Polyps don't normally hurt, but they often bleed – sometimes spontaneously, at other times because their surface is prodded during intercourse or with an inserted tampon: or when their stalk (pedicle) gets twisted and strangulated, cutting off the blood supply to the polyp which then dies and starts to bleed. Polyps can be avulsed (twisted off their stalks painlessly) in out-patients, but a D & C is usually carried out as well, to test for polyps or cancer in the womb.

CERVICAL CANCER

There are two quite different sets of circumstances to consider under this heading: early changes in cell cytology that can last for some years (cytology just means the study of cells or, as used here, the results of studying cells removed for the purpose of diagnosis); and invasive cervical cancer.

1. HOW IT STARTS

The membrane (epithelium) at and around the squamo-columnar junction undergoes marked changes under normal conditions: metaplasia (see above) converts 'ectopic' (displaced) columnar cells into squamous cells, by means of the multiplication of reserve cells found immediately below them. The result is layers or strata of epithelium called 'stratified squamous epithelium' (like the naturally occurring type).

Under this recently formed 'transitional zone', as it is called, tiny nooks or crypts that once acted as reservoirs for the mucus formed by the columnar cells, remain in the same state without undergoing metaplasia, and tend to get at least partially crowded out and buried by the overlying squamous epithelium. The mucus (in theory) gets secreted by minute holes in the new squamous cells, but blockages often develop, giving rise to retention cysts. These provide the only clue to metaplasia, visible to the naked eye. It is important because the transitional zone is where squamous carcinoma invariably originates. Cervical smears *must*, therefore, be taken from the whole area embracing the squamo-columnar junction, *and* just outside it, *and* wherever retention cysts can be seen (which may be a large area).

What happens, apparently, is that the activity involved in metaplasia renders the cells especially vulnerable to carcinogenic stimuli. The cells' nuclei are crammed with genetic material constantly undergoing division to replace worn-out cells, *and* engaged in the process of changing their very nature. Biological counsel for the defence would doubtless maintain that his clients sometimes got carried away and lost control, dividing too quickly under the evil influence of certain triggers, turning out badly (becoming malignant) in the process. Precedents to such cellular anarchy can be traced to other sites where different cell types meet, e.g. just inside the anus or back passage, and in the lower part of the foodpipe or oesophagus.

Dysplasia seen on a smear refers to multiplication and multilayering of cells, and abnormalities in the genetic material inside the cells' nuclei.

A diagnosis of cervical cancer is a possibility so dreadful to many women, that they avoid smears altogether. This is tragic because the premalignant changes smears can detect, can be easily and successfully treated before invasion of underlying structures occurs, while the disease is still confined to the surface membrane of squamous cells (95%) or glandular cells (5%).

2. VARIOUS STAGES

Degrees of dysplasia are staged according to their clinical implication (and appropriate treatment). Known as cervical intra-epithelial neoplasia (CIN), it is classified as stage 1, 2 or 3 according to whether it is mild, moderate or severe. Severe dysplasia (CIN 3), also called carcinoma in situ (literally, carcinoma or cancer confined to one particular place), is Stage 0 of the cancer of the cervix.

Microinvasive carcinoma, where invasion or an 'eating into' of underlying structures has *just* started on a 'micro' or cellular level, is accepted by international convention as stage Ia(i) of the cervical carcinoma scale which, thereafter, runs through stages Ib to IV. The criteria involve the extent to which the disease has invaded, first, the cervix itself, then the vagina and/or wall of the pelvis and/or bladder and other pelvic organs; and, finally, organs beyond the pelvis, including secondaries (deposits of cancer arising from the original site and spreading via the bloodstream and lymphatics) in distant body areas and organs.

If you can't remember any of the above and would rather not try, at least you now know why confusion reigned for so long before international standards of classification and treatment were reached. This, in turn, explains why there are so many different names for the same thing. Benefits of at least glossing over these details include: a lingering impression of the early, preinvasive stages when the chances of recovery are very high; and some familiarity with such terms as 'dysplasia', 'CIN', 'microinvasive', 'Stage 0', if you happen to hear them from GPs, nurses, consultants or their staff, or catch sight of them in your medical records. The screen of the surgery computer always seems to be seen by the patient whenever notes reveal difficult, misinterpretable or controversial results and remarks.

3. CAUSES

The most notable trigger is intercourse, especially at an early age. Links exist with low socio-economic status; early marriage; having lots of children; promiscuity; prostitution; and sexually-transmitted diseases. Sperm DNA (genetic material) is probably the carcinogen. Both the genital herpes virus (herpes virus type 2) and, even more, the papilloma virus giving rise to genital warts, are also blameworthy; and tobacco smoking is thought to increase the risks.

Cervical cancer is exceedingly rare in virgins, relatively common after the age of forty, quite often found in women aged 30 to 39, and increasingly in young women between 20–29 years. It typically causes bleeding after intercourse, which, as mentioned elsewhere because it simply cannot be said too often, is a symptom that you really must NEVER ignore.

4. CONSULTING A DOCTOR

Abnormal cervical smears – cause grief, heartache and anxiety, chiefly because they are poorly understood (i.e. inadequately explained to patients). The abnormalities include *inflammatory* changes and 'unsatisfactory smear'. The former is usually due to Trichomonas, thrush or some other infection. Severe changes approach the borderline with CIN. The effects of the genital herpes virus and the genital wart virus are easily identified, although the latter can be hard to tell apart from CIN. Inflammatory changes due to ageing membranes deprived of oestrogen are also common after the menopause.

An unsatisfactory smear – means that no diagnosis can be made because there are too few cells, too much blood or inflammatory debris, or some other technical error. The national average of smears that need to be repeated, is 8–10%.

Colposcopy – is a way of viewing the cervix by means of a special bivalve speculum. It allows laser treatment or a biopsy to be performed under anaesthesia. Mucus is wiped away and the cervix painted with iodine or acetic acid to show up abnormal tissue. This can sting a bit afterwards.

Colposcopy should be performed whenever CIN is found, except when infection or post-menopausal membrane changes are present, in which case treatment should be given and the smear repeated.

5. TREATMENT

Destruction of diseased tissue to a depth of 7 mm by diathermy (heat) or laser beams, has largely replaced cone biopsy in the treatment of CIN. Invasive cervical cancer is treated with radio-therapy and/or surgery. Chemotherapy has proved disappointing. Nuclear magnetic resonance imaging (NMR) can be used to visualise a cervical cancer and reliably define its volume. This can facilitate comparison between the results of surgery and radiotherapy which has been prob-lematic in the past. Here are the five year survival rates for invasive cervical cancer, irrespective of the method of treatment:

STAGE	SURVIVAL
Ia	around 100%
Ib	85–90%
IIa	70–75%
IIb	50–60%
III	30–35%
IV	up to 10%

Chapter Seven

The Premenstrual Syndrome

The premenstrual syndrome is a constellation of symptoms that affect many women before the start of their periods. Reading about them may have confused you, since up to 150 have been linked with the condition (Solgar's Training Digest, A Natural Food Trader Guide, Vol. 3, Issue 1: Solgar are a dietary supplement company). And almost everyone who writes about PMS, proposes different causes and cures.

PMS Symptoms

Physical
fluid retention
weight gain
bloating
breast pain
headaches
aching muscles
pelvic pain

Emotional
tension
irritability
depression
lethargy
poor concentration
aggression
low libido

reduced urine output	food craving
appetite changes	alcohol craving
sleep changes	poor emotional control
poor co-ordination	
fatigue	

A diary is the biggest help in establishing whether or not you are a PMS sufferer; note daily for two to three months how you feel, when (if) symptoms come on, and – just as importantly – when they stop. PMS is absolutely ALWAYS confined to the SECOND half of the cycle, starting anytime after ovulation and ending WITHIN ONE TO TWO DAYS of the start of the following period.

WHO SUFFERS?

Unlike period pains (see Chapter 3), PMS gets worse with age; so women in their 30s onwards suffer most. PMS can also co-exist, or become confused with, the menopause from the mid 40s onwards.

The numbers of women affected vary according to which studies you read. Solgar (see above) referred to 'as many as forty per cent of women seeking medical help to relieve their symptoms of premenstrual syndrome...'. In 'The Premenstrual

Syndrome – Curing the REAL Curse'[1], I say that all women are conscious of SOME physical and/or emotional change before their period, 25% barely notice anything at all, 50% notice moderately severe problems, and the remaining 25% have a proportion of their lives badly affected in consequence. My experience since, offers me no reason to change my mind.

Here is a table prepared by Dr. A C Stewart, Member of the Royal College of Physicians, with Maryon Stewart LDH and S Tooley SEN, three members of the Women's Nutritional Advisory Service which incorporates The Premenstrual Tension Advisory Service[2]. The table comes from the monthly medical journal *Maternal and Child Health*, March 1992, and summarises the numbers of women suffering from PMS, grouped according to severity.

The survey itself looked at certain dietary items believed to trigger premenstrual problems, e.g. caffeine, lack of fibre, as well as the amount of exercise taken by 389 readers of *Fitness* magazine:

	Severe	Moderate	Mild	Non-sufferer
No. of Significant PMS symptoms	7	3–6	1–2	None (!)
No. of women	142	142	73	32

[1] Published by Thorsons Ltd., first edition, 1983; second (revised) edition 1992.

[2] Located in Lewes, East Sussex BN7 2QN, tel. 0273 487366

| Mean age/years | 30.9 | 29.2 | 28.8 | 26.3 |
| % with children | 60 | 56 | 43 | 31 |

The next table by the same authors shows the prevalence of the various symptoms:

Irritability	74%	Abdominal bloating	42%
Mood swings	61%	Sweet cravings	42%
Depression	57%	Breast tenderness	39%
Fatigue	49%	Clumsiness	25%
Tension	45%	Headache	21%
Increased appetite	44%	Poor concentration	18%

Four of the five most prevalent symptoms are emotional, which fits in with other research findings and lots of anecdotal accounts, most of which indicate irritability, moodiness, aggression, weepiness, as the worst problems. Dr. Peter Moore's feature in the *Trainee* Section of *Pulse*, the weekly medical newspaper for GPs, (May 16, 1992), mentions 'numerous studies linking behavioural changes to the menstrual cycle', such as:

increased criminal tendency among women offenders;

men late for work more often when partner premenstrual;

women child-abusers more likely to repeat abuse then;

accidents commoner (related to physical clumsi-

ness and tiredness as well as tension, irritability
etc. – author);

attempted suicide commoner;

higher rates of absenteeism, and work performance deteriorates (no wonder women's self-
esteem falls, then – author);

agoraphobia commoner – avoidance of social
activities

For these reasons, some doctors and other health
experts have come to dismiss PMS, as either
imaginary or psychosomatic (physical problems
arising from psychological causes). In his influential best-seller 'Not All In The Mind', consultant
psychiatrist Dr. Richard McKarness described the
effects of both artificial additives *and* certain
nutrient deficiencies on behaviour, mood, and
mental diseases such as schizophrenia. The general view now lies somewhere between these
points.

CAUSES

Doctors and health experts agree about one thing
– the causes are '*multifactorial*', i.e. arising from or
triggered by more than one, and probably a whole
handful, of factors. Dr. Peter Moore's view is that
no-one is yet certain, but he mentions various

theories related to diet, our immediate surroundings and the environment generally, the sort of lives we lead, our personalities, and our hormonal and genetic makeup.

In particular, Dr. Moore says that the symptoms are probably due to ovarian-linked factors rather than to the menstrual cycle as a whole; and that progesterone deficiency has probably got nothing to do with premenstrual syndrome. This knocks on the head theories which were virtually religious dogma until quite recently. Dr. Moore says: 'progesterone treatment, although still very popular, is ineffective both in tablet and pessary form'.

1. PROGESTERONE AND LOW BLOOD SUGAR

The high priestess of progesterone therapy, Dr Katherina Dalton, now 75, was the first to link progesterone and low blood sugar as a cause. In fact, long before I became acquainted with PMS as a doctor, she treated me as a patient for about three months with Cyclogest – progesterone pessaries I used twice daily. At first, my main symptoms, depression and lethargy, responded well; but the effect grew less monthly until I was gaining no benefit at all.

Dr Dalton, still a somewhat awe-inspiring character, now explains that progesterone's usefulness is related to low blood sugar level (hypoglycaemia). A number of factors can cause this, including the fibre and/or refined sugar content of food, time of meals or snacks, and (especially) frequency of length *and* timing of gaps between meals.

Hypoglycaemia stimulates the 'fight or flight' adrenal glands, which make and release the hormone hydrocortisone to normalise the blood sugar level, until food is once again absorbed from the gut. This can interfere with the body's utilisation of progesterone, and PMS symptoms occur in some women.

A similar enigma is mentioned later in this chapter in connection with evening primrose oil, i.e. that symptoms mimicking those of progesterone deficiency develop although blood levels are normal.

2. MAGNESIUM DEFICIENCY

This is the most consistent abnormal finding, according to the Women's Nutritional Advisory Service. The low magnesium levels discovered in the red blood cells of PMS patients have been linked to the many roles this mineral plays throughout the body and in the menstrual cycle. Magnesium aids fat and carbohydrate metabolism, releases cellular energy, protects the bowel from a build-up of lead, and helps to make protein and new cells. This is especially important in women who have to rebuild their womb lining and replace shed blood monthly.

The following actions of magnesium are directly connected with the menstrual cycle:

prostaglandin production (magnesium is a vital co-factor in our use of essential fatty acid GLA – see below).
balancing body's fluid levels
regulating hormone manufacture and release
maintaining a healthy nervous system
aiding muscular action (link with fatigue and/or co-ordination?)
normalising blood sugar, and therefore energy, levels
reducing stress (known as anti-stress mineral)

Green leafy vegetables, fish, snails, nuts, soya foods and milk, molasses, citrus fruits, corn on the cob, sunflower seeds and cold-pressed seed and nut cooking oils, all supply magnesium. But deficiencies can arise if we crash diet or live on junk foods; drink too much alcohol; take combined oral contraceptives or some other form of synthetic oestrogen; or suffer from chronic wasting disease or severe burns.

3. PROSTAGLANDIN E1 DEFICIENCY
Prostaglandins – PGs – are short-lived, hormone-like body chemicals that exert second-by-second control over cellular processes throughout the

body. They are classified and named according to their functions; and a group known as PG E1 (prostaglandins of the E1 set) are especially important in regulating the menstrual cycle. Evening primrose oil's popularity as a safe, natural treatment for PMS ties in closely with PG E1 levels.

Studies carried out since the 'sixties' in more than 20 universities and hospitals throughout Europe, the US and Canada, have established that evening primrose oil (EPO) is the preferred source of supplementary GLA (gammalinolenic acid), an essential fatty acid without which the body cannot make PG E1s. Supplementary GLA overcomes a problem many of us have, of manufacturing (enough) GLA for ourselves. Though provided with the right 'internal environment' and the enzymes to carry out the process, using polyunsaturates in cold-pressed plant oils, (soft vegetable margarines etc.), we are prevented from making enough FLA by factors mostly beyond our control, e.g.

too much saturated animal fat in diet
ditto alcohol
use of superprocessed cooking oil (cis-linoleic acid loses much of its nutritional value when hydrogenated, heated to high temperatures, etc)

ageing process
viral infections
cancer
radiation
(prolonged) physical and/or emotional stress, since stress hormone adrenaline strongly opposes GLA manufacture.

These factors individually and collectively weaken or suppress the enzyme D-6-D (delta-6-desaturase) which converts GLA into prostaglandins E1. A shortage of PG E1s hypersensitises the body to minute fluctuations in sex-hormone chemistry, so that symptoms normally caused by high prolactin or low progesterone levels occur despite normal levels of both.

4. MALNUTRITION

We tend to associate malnutrition with starving populations in famine-stricken countries and with low-income Western families during a recession. But it means far more than starvation in the conventional sense. Many of us in Europe and the US suffer from obesity due to a superfluity of refined sugar snacks and junk foods, yet are still malnourished. We need daily intakes of a wide range of vitamins, minerals and trace elements like selenium, chromium, copper, simply to provide energy and ward off major illnesses and infections.

These requirements are catered for – inadequately, according to some prominent food scientists – by nutrient RDAs (Recommended Daily Allowances or Amounts) calculated by the WHO (World Health Organisation), COMA and various nutritional advisory boards in Amsterdam, for the EC, US and Britain.

Our nutritional needs, however, are greatly increased by lifestyle features such as aerobic exercise, slimming, heavy physical work, long hours, persistent stress, combined with personal poisons like heavy drinking, smoking, misuse of drugs and/or patent medicines, and illicit substance abuse. One cigarette, for example, destroys 25 mg of vitamin C, which the body cannot store anyway, since it is water-soluble and lost in urine. Abuse of laxatives (which means using them either for slimming purposes or for weeks or months on end for constipation), especially those, like senna, that work by irritating the bowel, can wash many nutrients out of the gut before it's had a chance to absorb them.

Illnesses such as Coeliac disease (sensitivity to protein gluten in wheat and many other cereal crops), gastroenteritis, chronic diarrhoea, ulcerative colitis, Crohn's disease (inflammation of the small bowel) and malabsorption syndromes have a similar effect. Very few people could claim that their diet met all their nutritional needs especially when these are further increased by menstruation and other physiological events such as pregnancy, breast-feeding, puberty, adolescence and ageing. Suspected links between generalised malnutrition (including specific deficiencies, e.g. zinc, magnesium, vitamin B6) and PMS, supported by research and personal experience, will be discussed further in the Treatment section.

TREATMENT

1. MEDICAL TREATMENT
(1) The combined oral contraceptive (birth pill combining oestrogen and progesterone) is occasionally prescribed for PMS. However, as Dr. Peter Moore mentions in the *Pulse* article referred to earlier, 'the only effective treatment in placebo-controlled trials are (sic) ones that totally suppress ovulation' and goes on to suggest that this is best achieved by an oestradiol (type of oestrogen) implant; or the transdermal (stick-on) skin patch.
(2) Dr Moore also mentions danazol (Danol) as 'highly effective (for PMS) if given in a large enough dose to stop periods'. Danazol suppresses the release of the pituitary hormones controlling ovulation and the menstrual cycle. And he recommends regular exercise and a low sugar and salt/high fibre diet.

(3) Diuretics (water pills) are helpful for troublesome water retention; and mefanamic acid (Ponstan – see Chapter 3), 500 mg three times daily, is useful if the course is started before the symptoms. PMS symptoms begin immediately after ovulation in some women, giving them symptoms for 14 days per cycle; while some sufferers feel unwell for only a day or two before their periods. However, they're usually predictable as they maintain a pattern in individual women. Short courses of low dose tranquillisers and/or counselling help to control irritability or violent tendencies. Incapacitating depression, even though brief, needs medical advice.

2. SELF-HELP/NATURAL REMEDIES
Diet. Here are the basic guidelines to healthy eating. There are hundreds of more detailed versions – wholefood manufacturers often supply free dietary and recipe leaflets, as do the free newsletters and newspapers available in health food shops.

It's vital to prioritise your personal tastes wherever you can. It would be pointless to condemn yourself to a future of super vitality breakfasts of unsweetened muesli, skimmed milk and fruit juice if all you can face, first thing, is hot buttered toast and black coffee. Continue as before, substituting wholegrain, granary or seed bread for white, and a polyunsaturate spread like Flora or Flora Light. Use real butter occasionally, to avoid feeling deprived.

Other standard advice: eat complex carbohydrate energy foods daily – wholegrain bread, flour and its products, pulses, whole cereals; and two portions of fresh fruit and vegetables. Cut down on salt (you can use a potassium-based substitute such as Lo-Salt) and sugar (you can replace it with honey, molasses, finely-chopped fresh or dry fruit or a synthetic sweetener). Avoid saturated animal fat, and use low fat equivalents, i.e. yoghourt, cheese, skimmed milk; poultry, fish and eggs for protein; and cold-pressed, polyunsaturated plant oils, e.g. olive, corn oil for cooking. Stir-frying, steaming, baking, grilling (and brief boiling for fresh veg), preserve more vitamins and minerals and use little fat, compared to roasting and conventional frying.

Hypoglycaemia – a 'customised' diet based on the above, should also help to stabilise your blood sugar. Rebecca Willis, whose PMS responded to Dr. Katherina Dalton's anti-hypoglycaemia plan, explained in a magazine article how this meant eating little and often – at least three hourly during the day – and within an hour of waking and less than an hour of going to sleep at night.

Dr. Dalton claims that her strategy has helped two thirds of her patients, especially those with eating disorders such as bulimia nervosa which can devastate blood sugar metabolism. Women need 'to graze', particularly on complex carbos like rice, potatoes, flour, rye and oats, which release glucose *slowly* into the bloodstream. Pasta, pizza, rice or oat cakes, crispbread, Westphalian rye bread, porridge and jacket potatoes are so filling, they are unlikely to prove fattening if you avoid adding butter, sour cream, fatty cheese or sauces.

A year into her three hour nibbling plan, Rebecca Willis still felt fragile and tearful before periods, but in control; and her symptoms had noticeably improved. Initially, changing her eating habits was a bind, but finally worthwhile.

Herbal remedies – PMS diuretics include – celery, parsley, parsley piert, asparagus. Agnus castus relieves a range of PMS symptoms.

Homeopathic remedies for PMS – Sepia, Mag-M (Magnesium muriatica or magnesium chloride) and Kreosotum (creosote) for irritability and tension. Breast tenderness can often be relieved with Calc. (Calcarea ostrearum – oyster shell) or Conium maculatum (poison hemlock).

Aromatherapy essences useful for PMS include: Chamomile (where there is poor sleep and nervous tension); rose or sandalwood (to lighten a mood and increase sexual desire). Marjoram, lavender or chamomile as a hot compress on the tummy, added to bathwater, or massaged in a carrier oil into the lower abdomen or back eases cramping pains. Rosemary and geranium also help to relieve bloating due to the fluid retention characteristic of PMS.

Chapter Eight

MENOPAUSE AND AFTERWARDS

We usually use 'menopause' – which means literally 'the end of menstruation' – to refer to the physical and emotional changes that mark the end of a woman's reproductive years, known medically as the climacteric. I will go on using 'menopause' in this way to avoid confusion.

HISTORY

Records show that the age at menarche (first period) has fallen progressively over the past 100 years, due to improved health standards, medical treatment and nutrition. The age at the menopause has in contrast risen, but over a much longer timespan: according to the Greek philosopher physicians Aristotle and Hippocrates, and contemporary Roman authors, women 2000 years ago became menopausal in their early forties. They also died much sooner than we do, which means that their reproductive lives were comparatively long – possibly nature's way of helping to compensate for the far higher numbers of babies who failed to survive their first year of life. Historical population studies of medieval Europe show an average menopausal age of around 50, and today, about 50% of women in industrialised Western cultures have had their last period by the age of 51.

FACTORS INFLUENCING MENOPAUSAL AGE

These have interested and perplexed women and doctors for decades. The age at menarche was once thought to be closely linked to menopause, some authorities maintaining that the earlier menstruation started, the longer it would last; and vice versa. This does not seem to be the case, although race, nutritional standards and parity (number of babies born) *are* influential.

Black South African and American women stop menstruating sooner than white women; studies in New Guinea, borne out by research elsewhere confirmed that severely-malnourished women with low height and weight bled for the last time aged 43.6 years on average, compared with better-nourished native women in the same region (normal height and weight) who did so at 47.3 years. Similarly, women who have never given birth tend to have an early menopause, while having several babies – especially for women in the higher socio-economic groups – predisposes to a later one.

A report in the British Medical Journal (June 1, 1991), also shows that mothers of twins go through the 'change' around a year earlier than mothers of singleton offspring. Age at the time of the final pregnancy may also play a part: women who give birth for the last time before the age of 28 tend to have an earlier menopause than those who have babies after that age.

We have much to learn about the menopause and its causes: according to the BMJ report, there is even some evidence that blindness may extend menstruation. Chronic infectious illnesses or pelvic and genital diseases may affect fertility but, with the exception of inflammation of the ovaries due to the mumps virus, they do not seem to bring on an earlier menopause. However, according to some research studies into the X (female sexual) chromosome, hereditary factors may play a part; and the influence of tobacco smoking has been confirmed in a number of studies. Women smokers experience the menopause up to two years earlier than non-smokers. Possible explanations based on laboratory studies include ovarian enzymes that convert hydrocarbon molecules in the smoke into chemicals that prematurely age or destroy potential egg cells (and predispose to cancer).

100

Egg Numbers

This brings us to the most important influence on menopausal age – the number of ovarian follicles, the specialised structures in the ovary in which egg (oocytes) ripen prior to ovulation.

Forerunners of 'proper' eggs called primitive germ cells in a female embryo enlarge and multiply to reach between five and seven million by the twentieth week of pregnancy. They then divide in such a way that each new egg contains half the adult complement of chromosomes (a prerequisite to uniting with a sperm, which also contains half the normal adult number). Each egg becomes surrounded by a single layer of flat cells, the two structures together constituting a primordial (primitive) follicle. No further multiplication is possible unless and until fertilization occurs, so the numbers of eggs can only fall. They are usually down to around 2 million in the newborn baby girl (one million per ovary), and around half a million at puberty.

We are, therefore, kitted out with a fair number of potential menstrual cycles before even reaching the menarche: yet in practice, fewer than 0.01% are ovulated. Of the 20 or so follicles that proceed to develop each cycle, only one actually makes it to maturity, probably by capturing and thereafter monopolising the available blood supply early on in the monthly development 'race'. (This does not explain why the maturing follicles degenerate in the *other* ovary, however, where the blood supply remains equally available for all of them.)

Numbers of ovarian follicles fall steadily until around the time of the menopause when, influenced by changing levels of pituitary and ovarian hormones, the process accelerates and the final period occurs when the follicles have reached a critical number.

The precise trigger to the accelerated loss of follicles is not yet known, nor have researchers discovered the part if any, played by higher centres in the brain acting on the pituitary gland through the medium of the hypothalamus.

A premature menopause is one that occurs before the age of 40. No explanation can be produced in about 90% of cases; but possibilities include immune disorders, and cancer treatment with chemotheraphy or radiotherapy.

THE MECHANISM: HOW PERIODS CEASE

Periods tend to come to an end in one of three ways. They can simply stop, a normal period one month never being repeated, so that you learn only retrospectively that you have started the change. Alternatively, your periods may be separated by increasingly long intervals before disappearing altogether. Thirdly, the amount of blood shed monthly can gradually diminish to the (logical) point at which you lose none at all. In practice, six months without menstrual bleeding are needed for the menopause to be recognised; even so, the remaining follicles in the ovaries can be sufficiently active to cause further bleeds up to a year after the 'final' period, and these can easily be confused with more worrying causes of postmenopausal bleeding.

CONTRACEPTION

Contraceptive advice for around the menopause includes using protection for at least one year after periods have stopped. Fertility declines from the mid-20s onwards and is greatly reduced after the age of 40: but the possibility of conceiving persists, although periods become at least partly anovulatory (occurring without ovulation) during the climacteric, a time when cycle length can also vary greatly. A link with reproductive age suggests that women who have a late menopause e.g. 55 years or older, tend to have longer cycles separated by longer intervals than women whose periods stop by the time they are 44.

FSH

As mentioned before, the variable factor(s) are associated with the first half (follicular phase) of the cycle between day one of a period and ovulation, when FSH (follicle stimulating hormone) is produced by the pituitary gland to ripen the follicles. The luteal phase between ovulation and the next blend, is by comparison far more constant, at around 14 days in most instances.

FSH (and LH) levels generally rise during the late 40s early 50s, suggesting a decrease in the follicles' sensitivity to FSH; and a redoubling of efforts on behalf of the hypothalamus to persuade the pituitary to get them to work. This negative feedback mechanism, i.e. the less responsive the follicles, the more FSH secreted, may be brought about partly by reduced levels of a hormone called inhibin (follicle stimulating release inhibiting substance), which is secreted during the fertile years to keep the manufacture and release of FSH under control. Whatever the explanation, anovulatory bleeding following a rise and fall in oestrogen levels without measurably increased progesterone levels, occur side by side with normal, ovulatory bleeding.

You can, therefore, expect your periods to show some irregularity before the menopause, while still sticking to one of the three common 'exit routes' mentioned, i.e. stop suddenly, get farther apart, or just more and more scanty. What you should watch out for, though, is complete irregularity, with days or weeks of heavy blood loss interspersed with unpredictably long or short non-bleeding intervals. The underlying problem needs to be determined, to rule out uterine cancer and other serious illnesses, none of which can clear up without diagnosis and treatment.

SYMPTOMS

It has been estimated that about 70% of women suffer some discomfort during the menopause. The main symptoms are:

Hot flushes and sweats
Lethargy
Anxiety, depression, irritability
Loss of confidence
Low libido (sexual desire)
Insomnia
Headaches
Poor memory and concentration
Vaginal dryness
Painful intercourse
Urinary symptoms
Accompanying skin and hair changes.

They are best understood in relation to the three main types of disturbance involved.

THREE MAIN TYPES OF DISTURBANCE

1. CIRCULATORY IMBALANCE

Hot flushes and night sweats (daytime sweats, too, which seem to be even worse) are probably caused by a menopausal-linked defect in the hypothalamus, which normally controls the calibre of the arterioles (tiny blood vessels supplying an area with blood) at the body's periphery. The arteries in the skin dilate, bringing the blood close to the surface, or become more narrow releasing or conserving heat as required.

Problems at central HQ (possibly connected with the high levels of circulating FSH) cause the vessels in the skin of the face, neck, chest and other areas, to dilate willy-nilly, producing a hot flush (or sweat). Another theory has it that vascular dilation coincides with a 'flushing band' of blood oestrogen levels peculiar to each woman, above and below which control is normal.

Whatever the explanation, affected areas become noticeably pinker, an event which can be highly embarrassing in public although people, generally, are so unobservant that flushes, sweats and other forms of suffering are a great deal less obvious than most of us believe. Night-time sweats are equally aggravating because they can lead to disturbed sleep, cold shivers and even necessitate several changes of nightwear and/or bedclothes during the course of a single night.

Flushes and sweats usually last for five to ten minutes, occur either rarely or several times in an hour, and are often accompanied by a racing pulse. Known medically as tachycardia, this symptom is frequently misdescribed as 'palpitations' by sufferers, who may then start to worry about heart disease as well as an uncomfortable change.

Flushes can be triggered by stress and anxiety, and physical factors such as a warm, stuffy atmosphere, alcohol, highly spiced food and strong tea and coffee. Similar triggers doubtless exist for night sweats, which are also aggravated by synthetic fibre bedclothing and nightwear. Simply changing to cotton or linen sheets, and pure cotton nightdresses or pyjamas can solve the problem more effectively than HRT, pills, potions, aromatherapy, meditation and the thousand and one other remedies 'experts' often rush forward to suggest.

2. MEMBRANE CHANGES

The membranous tissue lining the vagina and urethra (bladder outlet tube) age or degenerate as oestrogen levels fall, giving rise to a number of symptoms typical of the 'change'. Why should the urinary system be affected like the vagina? Because, in the developing embryo, a primitive structure called the Müllerian duct gives rise to the vaginal part of the bladder called the trigone, *and* the upper third of the urethra, so all three are influenced by oestrogen secretion.

The urethral syndrome, a common alternative diagnosis to true cystitis at any age (especially when no infection is present), produces a burning sensation on emptying the bladder (dysuria), increased frequency in passing urine, both during the day and at night, and sometimes even traces of blood in the water (haematurial). When the need to pass urine several times in the night is combined with night sweats, frustration, discomfort and fatigue it can, unsurprisingly, give you the screaming habdabs.

Other urinary symptoms during the menopause include urgency (having to reach a lavatory promptly to avoid an accident – urge incontinence), and stress incontinence – urine escaping when the pressure inside the abdomen (and therefore in and on the bladder) is raised. Triggers include coughing, sneezing, laughing, hiccuping, carrying heavy objects and straining to open the bowels. While not directly connected with low oestrogen levels, the weakening effects of the underlying contributory factors to stress incontinence – overweight, several pregnancies, long-standing cough, constipation – worsen as we age, ageing itself being accelerated in one way or another by hormonal changes throughout the body.

When the vaginal lining shrinks and grows old, penetrative sex can become excruciatingly painful. Firstly, the membrane's normal ridges and folds are lost, so the total area inside is diminished, reducing the available space and the flexibility of the vagina walls. Instead of the erect penis slipping easily into an elastic 'sac' which expands to its contours, it has to be forced into something resembling a plastic fingerstall, with practically no room for manoeuvre between walls with very little 'give'.

The consequent pain reduces the quantity of fluid secreted by the lubricating glands which, due to the fall in oestrogen, are in any case less productive. The vagina and vulva are often inflamed and sore because ageing membranes are unhealthy and more prone to infection (in this case from bacteria and/or yeasts such as thrush); and the pain and discomfort result from the combination of dryness, soreness and reduced room. The problem is self-perpetuating, because the anticipation of pain triggers anxiety, often with added emotional stress, and a form of vaginismus results, the lower pelvic and upper thigh muscles clamping down protectively to prevent entry. There's also the inherent loss of libido many menopausal women experience, unconnected with vaginal problems.

Obviously you'd have sex less often if you felt like this and, as with other underused organs, some women become less and less able to enjoy or even sustain love making. Interestingly, vaginal dryness and membrane degeneration are less pronounced in women who enjoy a regular and satisfactory love life.

Vaginal and urinary symptoms 'tend to occur...' some time after the inception of flushes and sweats. Later, the skin around the edges of the vulva and covering the labia majora (outer genital lips) becomes laxer and more obviously wrinkled. Severe vulval itching is common, and some women develop a condition known as kraurosis vulvae, in which the vulva becomes dry, painful and inflamed. Prompt treatment is needed to relieve the discomfort, prevent infections and reduce the slight risk of cancer later on.

3. PSYCHOLOGICAL DISTURBANCES
Women's unpredictable mood swings have become the butt of many jokes. Oestrogen levels are doubtless partly to blame – yet menopausal emotional problems tend not to respond to HRT in the absence of other symptoms, so the misery

must be partly caused by factors such as physical discomfort and insomnia.

Anecdotal evidence also suggests the importance of personality and lifestyle. Businesswomen and others with active interests outside the home and a positive attitude, apparently suffer less during the menopause than housewives who do not leave the home, especially those in lower income brackets. But this could equally mean different attitudes to HRT between social groups, and/or different nutritional standards.

The main emotional problems experienced during the 'change' are similar to those of PMS – irritability, sudden tearfulness, anxiety and a deepening loss of confidence, often aggravated by poor memory and concentration. It is tempting to oversimplify – to blame most if not all of these on the psychological challenges of ageing and becoming infertile.

Drooping breasts, wrinkles, hair loss, facial hair growth, weight gain, don't appear overnight, so we have time to get used to them; but no-one could deny their ability to undermine self-esteem and trigger anxiety and depression.

One form of depressive illness cannot be blamed upon other menopausal symptoms although it is probably aggravated by them. Some experts regard *involutional melancholia* (IM) as a form of depression that happens to coincide with

111

middleage (involution here means 'shrinkage of an organ'); others regard it as a discrete mental illness of people between the ages of 45 and 65. It affects women three times more often than men, and past emotional disorders are relatively rare although psychiatrists have identified what they term a premorbid personality, with a higher than average predisposition to 'obsessive compulsive traits'.

Involutional melancholia is a psychotic illness, meaning that sufferers experience some loss of contact with reality, generally in the form of delusional ideas about sin, guilt, worthlessness, poverty or disease. Some also feel depersonalised (that their body has changed in some way) or derealised (that their surroundings have altered and become subtly unfamiliar). Symptoms tend to develop gradually, and hypochondria is often the first to appear; concerns about the bowels being blocked are especially common. Many victims become restless, agitated and paranoid, i.e. feel persecuted, and dwell constantly on suicide and death (all melancholics are regarded as high suicide risks).

This illness requires professional medical treatment, with tricyclic antidepressants for mild to moderate IM, and ECT (electroconvulsive therapy) for severe symptoms, both of which are usually very successful. Self-help methods can be used to complement the effects, and will be dealt with later.

OSTEOPOROSIS

This refers to 'brittle bone disease'. The best way to conceptualize 'bone density' is as 'mass of bone per unit volume', e.g. number of grams of bone per cubic centimetre, or how much actual bony tissue – living cells, minerals calcium, magnesium, phosphorous etc – can be crammed into a small space.

Human bone is densest and therefore strongest during our mid-30s. Thereafter, old cells are broken down and resorbed more rapidly than they are reformed, and minerals leach out faster than they can be replaced. The bones remain roughly the same size in outline but there is a gradual loss of matrix (the main substance from which they are formed), plus loss of strengthening calcium with which the matrix is impregnated. Yearly loss can reach 2% of cortical bone (outer hard shell) and 7% of the spongy interior packing; put another way, by the time you're 70, you can have lost 50% of your total bone mass if you're female – by comparison, around 25% by the time you're 95, if you're male.

Osteoporosis affects around five million people in the UK, particularly postmenopausal women because bone destruction and mineral loss are accelerated by the fall in oestrogen (and also by rheumatoid arthritis and other conditions including overactivity of the thyroid gland – thyrotoxicosis, both of which are common in women – and overactive adrenal glands as in Cushing's disease).

Osteoporotic bones can become so porous and brittle that they splinter or snap following the simplest stress, e.g. a light fall or harmless act such as coughing. Fractured hip is notorious; besides costing the NHS more than £100m yearly, 15% of patients sustaining this injury die within three months, about 25% of patients die within a year, and 50% are never able to walk unaided again. Experts have estimated that around 50% of women aged 70 in the UK suffer a minimum of one osteoporotic fracture. Fractures of the spine and wrist are also common. Vertebral fractures are often spontaneous and, while some cause severe back pain, many are symptomless. Multiple fractures within the spinal column lead to loss of height, and also to Dowager's hump.

CONSULTING A DOCTOR

A choice of non-invasive methods now exist for measuring bone mineral density at typical fracture sites; the National Osteoporosis Society provides details of local facilities in response to written enquiries (PO Box 10, Radstock, Bath BA7 3YB).

Bone densitometry costs about £86 and should be repeated yearly if a positive diagnosis is made. Other tests include X-rays, usually following a fracture, pain or other symptoms; blood tests, including calcium levels; and tests of liver and thyroid function.

Most GPs treat osteoporosis themselves, referring to hospital only patients who appear to have some complication or whose symptoms need further explanation in view of their age or other health factor. HRT can greatly reduce bone loss; and established risk factors can be replaced by healthy habits to aid prevention. Useful tips include a balanced diet based on natural, whole foods; controlled alcohol intake; not smoking; and regular weight-bearing exercise e.g. brisk walking, dancing, trampolining, and jogging.

Other forms of aerobic exercise improve overall fitness but do not strengthen bones nor help to increase bone mass (i.e. drive calcium from the bloodstream into the skeleton). This finding followed tests on astronauts during American space mission training, when the bones of volunteers were found to lose significant amounts of calcium during flights when their feet lacked contact with hard surfaces due to the absence of gravity.

Promotional campaigns by pharmaceutical companies and health authorities have emphasised modern HRT's effectiveness and safety, and it is now prescribed more widely than it was ten years ago. Interest in self-help methods continues to grow, however, especially among women for whom supplementary oestrogen is unsuitable. A balanced diet, exercise (and relaxation), and a 'healthy habits' routine regarding alcohol and cigarettes have already been mentioned.

AFTER THE MENOPAUSE

You may not expect a book entitled *Problem Periods* to offer several thousand words on the menopause, a time when, logically, menstrual problems ought no longer to exist. Apparently haphazard meanderings around the realm of post-menstrual disorders might seem even less directional. Yet two female genital cancers pose such serious threats to middle-aged and older women, advantage should be taken of every opportunity to describe and explain their warning signs.

1. UTERINE CANCER
This affects the lining of the uterus or endometrium, hence its medical name of endometrial carcinoma. It gives rise to (often heavy) vaginal bleeding around the time of the menopause, post-menopausal bleeding thereafter, and often a brown, watery offensive discharge.

116

Obesity and diabetes are both risk factors, but weight reduction and blood glucose control reduce this extra risk to around normal.

About 15% of patients experience tummy pain thought to be caused by expulsive uterine contractions stimulated by the malignant cells within. The commonest discomfort sites include the upper, central part of the abdomen between the down sweep of the lower ribs (the hypogastrium); and the right or left lower abdominal quadrants, i.e. over the appendix and the corresponding area on the left, known medically as the iliac forrae.

There is an increase in endometrial cancer because women, in common with the population at large, are living longer and hence are around to contract the disease.

2. CANCER OF THE OVARIES

Cancer of the ovaries is slightly commoner than endometrial cancer (rates per 100,000 population of newly diagnosed cases, around 13.0 and 16.5 respectively) but, like endometrial cancer, it is a disease of the late 50s and 60s, and is notorious for 'silently' developing, causing symptoms too late for successful treatment.

There are more cases of ovarian cancer nowadays, probably because we live longer, and it has become the commonest fatal gynaecological malignancy, and one of the commonest of all cancers, in women. Approximately 20% of cell malignant growths in the ovary are 'secondaries' arising from a malignant primary tumour, typically, in the breast, stomach, colon, uterus, Fallopian tubes or the opposite ovary.

Early in the disease, vague symptoms like unexplained weight loss and tummy bloating may occur; these, and others such as tummy pains, indigestion, vomiting, passing urine more frequently and/or swollen ankles, appearing for the first time for no apparent reason, always require investigation. Later, severe weight loss with visible wasting (known as cachexia), fluid in the tummy cavity (ascites), pain in the lower back or pelvis, and, possibly, post-menopausal bleeding, can all be experienced.

Factors believed to increase the chances of contracting this cancer include: late childbearing, lowgrade infertility, irradiation, the blood group A, anticonvulsant drugs, incessant ovulation (which helps to explain the partial protection provided by childbearing and oral contraceptives), and exposure to asbestos and/or talc. Most people are aware of the dangers of asbestosis, a lung complaint unprotected asbestos workers often develop and which predisposes to cancer. Talc, a relatively soft, greasy mineral compound of magnesium and silica, is the major component of soapstone (stearite) and, besides being made into talcum powder, is also used as an industrial filler, lubricant and soft abrasive.

3. CONSULTING A DOCTOR
Make sure you have worrying symptoms investigated, even though patients (and GPs) currently have an allotted five minutes of consultation time per visit. This may mean being more assertive with your doctor than you normally are, or just braving it and 'making a nuisance of yourself'. Pre-operative investigations may include: a cervical smear; full blood count and ESR (erthrocyte sedimentation rate – the rate at which the red cells in a sample of blood form a sediment at the bottom of a measuring tube); other blood tests, e.g. levels of various minerals or 'electrolytes' (for instance, potassium, sodium), and of urea (which reflects kidney function); liver function tests; MSU – midstream urine specimen (generally reveals urinary infection if present); intravenous urogram (major test of kidney and bladder function, showing images of the urinary tract on screen after injecting an intravenous dye); a lymphangiogram – contrast (dye-based) X-ray of lymph nodes and lymph ducts to reveal glandular involvement if present; chest X-ray; plain abdominal X-ray; paracentesis – examination of cellular content of excess fluid or ascites, withdrawn from abdominal cavity; barium enema; ultrasound.

The prime object is to identify an ovarian tumour if present, after ruling out other causes of the symptoms. Common examples of the latter include fibroids; obesity; cysts (bloating); appendix abscess (tummy pain); diseased or aberrant kidney e.g. a kidney that has developed in the pelvis rather than higher up (urinary problems); infection or fluid swelling of the Fallopian tubes (feeling generally unwell); diverticulitis – a common bowel complaint; a distended bladder arising for some other reason (difficulty passing urine); and tumour(s) of the broad ligament(s) supporting the uterus, the colon, rectum or another pelvic organ (weight loss, bloating, general ill health).

4. TREATMENT

The prime aim of operating is the removal of the uterus, ovaries and tubes; the secondary aim is to enable the surgeon to assess the extent of the disease and biopsy suspicious areas.

Ovarian cancer is classified as stage 1–4 in ascending order of severity, from a simple (stage 1), well-differentiated tumour confined to the ovary, unaccompanied by ascites – abdominal fluid – which may be successfully treated by surgery alone; through stages 2, 3 and 4 where the growth is very advanced and has involved other organs and tissues. Stage 2 is treated by surgery and radiotherapy, and possibly cytotoxic drugs to kill the malignant cells; stage 3 is generally treated with surgery and chemotheraphy only; and chemotherapy alone tends to be prescribed for very advanced states (stage 4).

TREATMENT

1. MEDICAL

Medical treatment for menopausal symptoms is mainly by HRT (see Chapter 9). However, an alternative is tibolone.

Tibolone (Livial) 'appears to be an ideal drug for the menopausal woman who still has a uterus and has no desire to experience monthly withdrawal bleeding' (consultant gynaecologist Janice Rymer in *The Journal of Sexual Health* June/July 1992).

Chemically similar in structure to naturally occurring hormones, synthetic tibolone behaves like a weak oestrogen and progestogen, and a very weak androgen. It is proving a popular alternative to conventional HRT for the relief of post-menopausal symptoms, especially (according to double-blind, placebo-controlled studies) hot flushes, insomnia, depression, low sex drive, vaginal dryness and painful intercourse.

Tibolone has no adverse effects on blood pressure, the endometrium (lining of the uterus) or bone density (it may help to prevent further bone loss and even increase bone density in women with diagnosed osteoporosis). It doesn't appear to be harmful to the heart or circulation, although it decreases levels of protective HDL cholesterol. Its weak hormonal action suggests benefits for menopausal women with histories of breast or endometrial cancer, or who have undergone a pelvic clearance operation for endometriosis (any remaining deposits of endometrium are less likely to bleed with tibolone than with HRT).

Tibolone is taken by mouth in a single 2.5 mg daily dose. If you have been on conventional HRT and want to change, you would either be swapped straight over or given supplemental progestogen for the last 12 days of the first month's treatment. Withdrawal bleeding, should it occur, is usually due to previous HRT or your own oestrogen production. You can either change back to HRT after three months or continue to take additional progestogen until the bleeding stops. Tibolone by itself can also cause break-through bleeding for the first four to six months.

2. NATURAL REMEDIES

Herbal remedies: helonias root works well as an ovarian and general menopausal tonic; good restoratives (which help to minimise the effects of hormonal fluctuations and of reduced oestrogen output), are St. John's wort, Agnus castus, life root and oats. If stress and irritability, tearfulness and tension bother you, try chamomile or black haw.

Damiana, saw palmetto, sarsaparilla, licorice, Agnus castus, ginseng may all help to improve a flagging sexual interest.

Homoeopathic remedies: Graphites, Sepia and Lachesis (Surukuku snake venom) can all help generally with menopausal problems. Sepia is especially indicated if you are feeling irritable. For irregular menses around the time of the menopause, Nit. Ac. (nitric acid) may be useful.

Aromatherapy: rose can increase feminine self-confidence and dispel doubts about personal sexual attractiveness. Both geranium and rose can ease general menopausal symptoms. Chamomile eases irritability. Other active anti-depressants include sandalwood, ylang-ylang, bergamot, clary sage, jasmine, lavender and neroli.

Chapter Nine

THE PILL AND HRT

I am dealing with the Pill and HRT in a separate chapter because female complaints are so often cured by them. They worry women particularly because of the short and long-term effects which the use of these chemicals may have – especially if taken over a period of years.

THE PILL

Oral contraceptives – OCs – received bad publicity in the 1970s, and are still avoided by women whom they would help because of possible side effects, particularly 'clotting of the blood'. But modern versions of the Pill with less oestrogen and newer progesterones, offer excellent contraceptive protection *and* medical benefits of which you should at least be aware. OCs can be chosen to suit individual patient's needs, e.g. the relief of breast tenderness, premenstrual acne, other PMS symptoms, period pain and irregular or heavy bleeding.

Neither doctors nor patients always get it right first time; the GP may choose an inappropriate COC (combined OC) due to individual bias or lack of experience, while any woman may forget to mention all her menstrual symptoms. But, as GP Martyn Walling explains in an article in a 1992 issue of the British Journal of Sexual Medicine: '...when the client returns with side effects after three cycles, it is then almost always possible to find the appropriate pill'.

1. SIDE EFFECTS

Side effects aren't inevitable; but examples of those that might occur include: breast enlargement, bloating with fluid retention, cramps and pain in the legs, loss of sexual desire, depression, nausea, vaginal discharge and breakthrough bleeding.

Reasons for immediately discontinuing treatment include: occurrence of migraine-type headaches for the first time, or frequent severe headaches; visual disturbances (non-specific, probably blurring, flickering lights etc); clotting of blood inside veins, with inflammation (thrombophlebitis), or clots, fragmenting within veins and entering the circulation (thromboembolism); rise in blood pressure; jaundice; pregnancy; six weeks before a major elective operation and during bedrest convalescence afterwards (because of risk of thrombosis although it can be taken again two weeks after the patient is fully mobile). This last point does not apply for minor operations with a brief anaesthetic, when the patient will soon be up and about, except minor procedures to the legs (e.g. resetting a fracture, bunion removal). When it is not possible to discontinue use before a major operation doctors often guard against the risks of thrombosis by giving a preventive (prophylactic) low dose injection under the skin, of an anticoagulant such as heparin.

2. BENEFITS

(1) reduced menstrual bleeding. In a prospective long-term study by the Royal College of General Practitioners (RCGP), begun in 1968, the cases of menorrhagia (heavy bleeding), irregular bleeding and intermenstrual bleeding were halved by COCs; and the incidence of iron deficiency anaemia was also significantly reduced.

(2) relief of period pain (dysmenorrhoea); research generally has shown this. The RCGP study showed a significant reduction in the number of cases of dysmenorrhoea: 3.8% per 1000 women-years, compared to 10.43% per 1000 women-years among non-users.

(3) less chance of fibroids – Oxford Family Planning Association (OFPA) long-term follow-up study showed a 17% reduction in incidence for each five years the Pill was used.

(4) less chance of ovarian cysts (65% reduction in incidence, according to the RCGP study; the OFPA study found a 49–78% reduction, depending upon the type of cyst involved).

(5) less chance of benign breast disease (50–75% reduced risk, compared with non-COC users, according to numerous studies).

(6) less chance of pelvic inflammatory disease (PID); risk cut by about 50%, plus a favourable influence on the course of the disease – Pill users less often affected by severe forms, according to a report in the American Journal of Obstetrics and Gynaecology, 1977).

(7) less chance of certain cancers: e.g. risk of developing *ovarian cancer* (fourth commonest cause of female cancer deaths) is 30–69% lower, according to various studies since 1977. Endometrial (womb) cancer, the third commonest, is significantly reduced in women over 40, although not in those under 40 (in which age group it is comparatively rare, anyway). The Pill has to be 'combined', not the sequential sort that provides first, oestrogen by itself, then progestogen, during the cycle. It is the progestogen that exerts the protective effect.

(8) advantageous blood lipid (fat) changes. Oestrogens reduce levels of harmful LDL (low density lipoprotein) cholesterol that contributes to arterial disease, coronaries and strokes; and

increase protective HDL (high density lipoprotein) cholesterol that has the opposite effect. Progestogens' influence on cholesterol varies; the newer ones, in the main, act favorably.

(9) less chance of thyroid disease and rheumatoid arthritis (RA). Studies show that both diseases are less common in oral contraceptive users. The RCGP study showed a 50% reduction in RA and, although more recent case control studies have not borne this out, oral contraceptives are known to increase blood levels of immunosuppressive body chemicals also found in increased amounts during pregnancy, when natural remissions of RA are particularly common.

(10) Oestrogen-dominant OCs in which the main effect comes from the oestrogen component, include: Brevinor, Marvelon, Ovysmen, Dianette and Mercilon, and they are most useful for progestogenic menstrual symptoms such as:

loss of libido (sex drive)
lassitude
depression
vaginal dryness
acne
oily hair and skin
amenorrhoea (loss of periods)
weight gain

Progesterone-dominant OCs include Loestrin 30, Ovranette, Microgynon 30, Eugynon 30; they relieve oestrogen-mediated period problems such as:

nausea
dizziness
breast tenderness
fluid retention
vaginal discharge
period pain
breakthrough bleeding (late cycle)
headaches

3. COCs AND OLDER WOMEN

If you are a non-smoker, healthy and in your 40s, you can safely continue to take COCs until the menopause, according to much modern thinking on the subject. Appropriate choices usually contain the newer progestogens that have no adverse effects on cholesterol levels, such as norgestimate (Cilest), gestodene (Femodene, Minulet) and desogestrel (Marvelon, Mercilon). Remaining on the Pill masks the menopause and, at the age of 50, you would be advised to stop taking it and use barrier methods for six months. If your periods return, the advice is to continue with the sheath, or cap until menstruation really has stopped, and HRT can be prescribed, if necessary.

The reasons for swapping is that the natural oestrogen in HRT controls menopausal symptoms better than the synthetic ethinyl-oestradiol in COCs.

4. AFTER GIVING BIRTH...

The old practice of starting women on the Pill before they leave hospital after having a baby, was discontinued because blood clotting factors and the risks of thrombosis do not return to normal until three to four weeks after delivery. COCs also tend to reduce the output and fat content of breast milk. If you do not breastfeed, you may start ovulating as early as four weeks after your baby is born.

You should either be given a prescription for a combined oral contraceptive at your routine postnatal check (carried out four rather than six weeks after delivery), or use some other type of contraceptive to make sure you do not fall pregnant again immediately. Spermicidals and barrier methods are usually adequate since the chances of conceiving, though very real, are lower than usual at this time.

5. CAN YOU TAKE THE PILL?

There are very few medical conditions where injectable hormonal contraceptives or progestogen-only Pills cannot be prescribed; and the list of contraindications to COCs is diminishing steadily because of their new, improved formulae. Currently still on this list are disorders that predispose to arterial disease, a family history of blood clotting malfunction with increased risk of thrombosis, liver ailments (until tests show a return to normal of at least three months), and breast cancer. Nowadays, COCs can be safely taken in some instances if you are a diabetic, providing you do not have concomitant disease of the retina, arteries or kidneys; and also if you suffer from essential hypertension (the commonest kind of high blood pressure), so long as treatment reduces it successfully to 160/90 mm mercury or less.

6. OESTROGEN AND PERIOD MIGRAINE

'The effects are amazing. Women come back and kiss you!' said consultant neurologist Dr. Franco Clifford-Rose, chairman of the Migraine Trust, in a recent article advocating supplementary oestrogen for women with regular periods and true menstrual migraine.

This is defined as migraine occurring on the day of onset of the period, plus or minus a day or so. Dr. Clifford-Rose said sufferers benefit from wearing an oestradial skin patch for three days immediately before their periods. Absorption of the hormone prevents the fall in blood levels which can trigger a migraine attack. He recommends that

GPs prescribe a 25 microgram patch initially, increasing the dose to 50 or 100 micrograms the following month if there is no response. Breast tenderness is the only real side effect. A patient information leaflet on oestrogen skin patches is available from the Migraine Trust, 45 Great Ormond Street, London WC1N 3HZ, tel. (071) 278 2676.

Hormone Replacement Therapy (HRT)

This vexed subject could easily justify a whole book, never mind a few pages of one chapter. So many different things are said about hormone replacement therapy that it is difficult to know what to believe; we normally end up believing what we subconsciously need to believe about controversial subjects, anyway, and no amount of research or erudite argument is going to alter this.

The principle underlying hormone replacement therapy is simple: supplementary oestrogen boosts declining levels in the body, relieving menopausal symptoms (see Chapter 8) and helping to prevent cardiovascular (heart and arterial) disease and brittle bones (osteoporosis). Early preparations, containing oestrogen alone, were found in some studies to increase the risks of endometrial (womb) cancer. Today, oestrogen is prescribed with

132

progesterone, 'opposed oestrogen therapy', which actually reduces endometrial cancer risks *below* average. In the main, GPs and gynaecologists recognise these benefits; but HRT does not, as yet, enjoy universal approval, as extracts from recent papers and research studies show.

1. RECENT RESEARCH STUDY FINDINGS

(1) GP Reactions. *Postal questionnaires* were sent to 1268 GPs throughout the UK, in a survey of prescribing habits and attitudes to HRT by the Medical Research Council (MRC) Epidemiology and Medical Care Unit at Northwick Park Hospital, Harrow, Middlesex. The 85% of (1081) of doctors in 220 (95%) practices who responded, were prescribing HRT to an estimated 9% of their female patients aged 40–64, and 55% were prescribing opposed oestrogen therapy to more patients than a year earlier.

More than half would consider prescribing HRT to prevent osteoporosis (62%) and cardiovascular diseases (57%) to women without menstrual symptoms. Overall, 79% of the doctors would definitely or probably consider entering women who had had a hysterectomy into a (randomised controlled) trial that compared 'unopposed' (oestrogen only) HRT with the combined sort, 49% would enter patients with a uterus into such a trial. And in a subsample, 85% (180 out of 210) would consider entering patients without menopausal symptoms into a trial comparing HRT with no treatment (unopposed in patients who had had a hysterectomy, opposed in those who had not).

The conclusion drawn by this survey's organisers, H C Wilkes MRC, scientific staff, and J W Meade, Fellow of the Royal College of Physicians and Unit Director, was that there is considerable uncertainty among general practitioners as to the balance of beneficial and harmful effects of hormone replacement therapy in the long term, particularly relating to its use in preventing osteoporosis and cardiovascular disease. 'Most doctors would be prepared to participate in ... trials to determine the long term effects of this increasingly widely used treatment' (British Medical Journal (BMJ), June 1, 1991).

(2) BMJ According to a paper in the Journal of Clinical Pathology summarised in the BMJ, November 14, 1992, two recent surveys had found that 'the effects of the menopause on women are poorly understood and inadequately treated'. One survey explored British companies' knowledge of, and provision for, the effects of the menopause. It revealed that fewer than 10% of the 168 companies, (chosen at random from,

among others, construction, manufacturing and service industries), had a formal policy on the issue and 40% of the personnel departments surveyed, were unaware that reduced productivity, fainting spells and memory lapses are menopausal symptoms. Half the companies had no nurse or doctor on site at least once a week, and 43% of those with a turnover in excess of £50 m admitted that they did not provide this facility for their staff.

Mr. Malcolm Whitehead, a consultant gynaecologist at King's College Hospital, London, commented in relation to this survey: 'Menopausal symptoms ... impair the concentration of all women. You don't have to be a high flier to be made miserable by the menopause'. (Very true; but I must comment here that, while menopausal symptoms doubtless impair concentration, not all women suffer from such symptoms.)

The second survey by the Amarant Trust, an independent charity seeking to broaden understanding of the menopause and HRT, found that 80% of the 3000 women felt that their GP had spent too little time with them at their first consultation for HRT (less than ten minutes in nearly 50% of instances). Just over half of the respondents had been treated by their general practitioner.

HRT clinics cost £15–£20 an hour, and many GPs cannot afford to run them. As many as 137 of the women in the Amarant Trust survey, with an intact womb were taking unopposed oestrogen, thereby running an increased risk of endometrial cancer. Only 11% of the women surveyed, expressed concern about taking HRT, but 62% of them were worried about the risk of breast cancer.

(3) GP News. The Weekly *GP News* provides a most useful page – 'Patient Reading' – to keep family doctors abreast of health articles in the popular end women's press. On February 5, 1993, the leading column dealt with a piece in that month's *Marie Claire* which 'would worry readers on HRT because it told them that they were at risk from breast cancer'. And 'A second article twists the knife, saying HRT makes the cancer more difficult to diagnose'.

Mr. Nigel Sacks, a consultant surgeon and breast expert at the Royal Marsden, believed the *Marie Claire* article was misleading. He said: 'Short term HRT – up to ten years' continuous use does not increase the risk of breast cancer. Over ten years it may increase the risk by up to 20%, but that is not proven. There is still concern about the risks in women with a strong family history of breast cancer, but the positive effects of HRT are well proven and should not be forgotten.'

Mr. Sacks discounted anxieties about detecting breast cancer, since mammogram techniques can compensate for the increased tissue density that results from HRT. He said that combined HRT may slow down the growth of breast cells, as well as protecting the uterus.

Another article in *GP* encourages GPs to give HRT to women with a high risk of breast cancer, including those who have already suffered from it: the argument is that HRT relieves menopausal symptoms that are making women's lives a misery (plus guarding against heart and bone disease), while a high cancer risk remains whether they take HRT or not. Mr. Sacks is quoted again here: 'There is no evidence from the literature (i.e. studies) that HRT is harmful for women at risk of breast cancer... (it) is still officially a contraindication for HRT, and I suggest it should be reserved for women with severe menopausal symptoms. Give these women the minimal dose for up to a year'. Mr. Malcolm Whitehead is also quoted here, to the effect that he is unconvinced that HRT has any adverse effect beyond that which is inherited, but advises GPs to try other solutions for menopausal symptoms first.

The introduction of a genetic test for breast cancer may lead not only to thousands of women receiving prophylactic (preventive) treatment with the antioestrogenic drug tamoxifen, but also help to solve the conundrum for some doctors respecting the prescription of HRT (although some experts are bound to disagree with one another, as more evidence for and against continues to come to light).

Women with a family history of breast cancer will be advised to have the test, which will initially be available at major research centres. Only one in 10 of the 24,000 women newly diagnosed in Britain each year are likely to carry the gene. Women who are gene carriers and haven't yet developed breast cancer have an 80% to 90% chance of contracting the disease.

Professor Goden McVie, the Cancer Research Campaign's scientific director, told MIMS (Medical Index of Monthly Specialists) Magazine Weekly, (7 December 1993): 'My best guess is that the gene ... will be located in 1994. We already have good probes near the gene'. Professor McVie said a test for the gene may well be available by the end of 1994.

(4) The Lancet. What about other HRT downsides? An article in *The Times* (February 1, 1992) by their health services correspondent, Jeremy Laurance, refers to the *Lancet* which claims that supplementary oestrogen has all the hallmarks of

an addictive drug, and that HRT may be as addictive as heroine or cocaine. Oestrogen lifts the mood and increases the feeling of well being. Some women return for repeat treatments at shorter intervals (indicating dependence), while others require increasing doses to maintain the effect or relieve withdrawal symptoms (suggesting tolerance). Oestrogen's reputation as a 'fountain of youth' compels some women to request HRT. The report's authors suggest caution in prescribing, but Mr. John Studd, consultant gynaecologist at King's College Hospital, says women need not worry: 'It may just mean they are addicted to feeling better'. High levels, he stresses, are good for depression and bones. But, he said, there was still a question mark over its role in breast cancer and the side effect of uterine bleeding.

2. MY OWN VIEWS

Most of the papers I have on HRT agree that only 10–15% of eligible women actually take HRT, and that a third of these abandon it within six months (four out of five without consulting their GP). Fear, lack of information, troublesome side effects and disappointed expectations of heightened sexuality, are all responsible. *Two out of three* of the 1000 women taking part in a national opinion poll reported in *Doctor* weekly newspaper (9 July, 1992) had no idea why the menopause happened, and a quarter of those who had never taken HRT, said it was going against nature.

In the same study, only 33% of the women knew HRT could help prevent brittle bone disease, and a tiny 3% mentioned the risk of heart disease as a motivation for taking it. The main side effects reported, mimicked the premenstrual syndrome, e.g. depression, anxiety, breast tenderness, bloating and pelvic cramps. Heavy or irregular bleeding can also prove troublesome; but most adverse symptoms can be relieved or eliminated by switching to an alternative preparation after three months.

My personal view is, don't *expect* to have menopausal problems; if you do get them, try natural remedies. If they don't work and HRT is suitable for you – give it a go.

3. CUSTOMISING HRT

Dr. Kevin Gangar, senior lecturer at St. Mary's Hospital, London, commenting on the above survey, pointed out that there are more than 20 varieties of HRT currently available, including tablets, surgical implants, skin patches containing both oestrogen and progestogen, creams and pessaries, so GPs can tailor treatment. He said: 'HRT is not just a packet of pills, it's as individual as having a shoe or a dress fitted'.

(1) Oestrogen implants. Implants are the best

way of ensuring a woman remains on HRT, but they have to be inserted under aseptic conditions and, once in place, they're hard to remove. Other problems include the possibility of infection, extrusion of the pellet, sometimes a surge of oestrogenic side effects, and the need to (remember to) take progestogen tablets which can cause vaginal bleeding and other symptoms, on certain days each month.

Implants are a common first choice after a hysterectomy, and a viable alternative for women who have suffered side effects from other preparations.

(2) The patch. But many GPs favour the combination patch because it is simple to use and side effects are few; although it can come off in water or irritate sensitive skin[1].

The chief advantages of skin patch administration were discussed in the British Journal of Sexual Medicine, May/June 1993. Oral HRT produces peaks and troughs in hormone levels, and a 'kick up the liver' (!!!) that can disturb fat and carbohydrate metabolism, and the blood's clotting mechanisms. Transdermal HRT was developed to avoid these effects and get the native hormone oestradiol into the circulation, achieving a sustained level and mimicking the premenopausal hormone status.

[1] Dr Carol Lole-Harris, *Pulse*, December 19–26, 1992

141

(3) Oral tablet. This also retains the beneficial effects of oral HRT on blood fat in relation to heart disease, i.e. it reduces levels of harmful LDL (low density lipoprotein) cholesterol, and increases those of protective HDL (high density lipoprotein) cholesterol. It even goes a step further, more effectively lowering blood levels of fatty triglycerides, and raising those of the specially useful HDL2 (independent risk factors for coronary heart disease in women).

New research to be published shortly will also show that, whereas HRT in tablet form can upset the balance of insulin (reducing glucose tolerance and predisposing to diabetes), transdermal (skin patch) HRT has no such effect.

4. HRT BEFORE MENOPAUSAL AGE

Younger women who have undergone the menopause before the age of 40, either spontaneously or following an operation to remove their ovaries, need relatively high doses of oestrogen to protect their bones, hearts and arteries, and may be prescribed a 50mg oestradiol implant, or a 100 microgram (Estraderm) patch.

In a recent study at St. Mary's Hospital mentioned in *The Practitioner*, April 1993, women in this group needed an average of three to four changes of treatment before the results were acceptable; and some needed as many as seven.

142

They also needed supplementary testosterone, (the ovaries secrete 'male' androgens which contribute greatly to both libido and physical and emotional well being). Supplementary testosterone is also useful for some women whose menopausal symptoms are well controlled by HRT but still lack sex drive.[2]

5. PROBLEMS ENCOUNTERED GETTING THE HRT RIGHT

For the 'average' woman the two commonest problems requiring customising care include progestogen side effects and heavy withdrawal bleeding. Breakthrough and irregular bleeding tend to affect 'perimenopausal' women who begin HRT for menopausal symptoms before their periods stop. Progestogens taken at the 'right' time in the cycle can help synchronise progestogen-triggered bleeding with menstrual blood loss. Standard preparations include Trisequens and Prempak-C.

Older women in their late 50s and 60s who wish for the benefits of HRT, need to be introduced to supplementary oestrogen very gradually since they have usually lacked this hormone for a long time, and a sudden onrush into the bloodstream can

[2] (Said) Kevin Gangar, Lecturer in Obstetrics and Gynaecology at St Mary's Hospital, London; and Elizabeth Kew, Research Sister, Menopause Clinic, King's College Hospital, London.

cause distressing breast tenderness, nausea, and heavy, painful bleeding.

One milligram of oestradiol, such as Climogest, or the Estraderm TTS 25 (mg) patch, may be suitable, together with counselling and information about side effects. A continuous course of progestogen such as Provera 5 mg might be added to the small oestrogen dose to stop monthly bleeds (this works best in older women, who are long past their last natural period). Long-term effects on the womb lining are still uncertain with currently available preparations, and it is recommended that these patients have an endometrial biopsy every 12–18 months while receiving this treatment.

6. OTHER USES OF HRT

Doctors sometimes prescribe HRT for troublesome conditions unaccompanied by other menopausal symptoms. It can help to relieve arthritis, muscular aches and pains, lethargy, hair loss, skin wrinkles, and poor concentration.

Chapter Ten

NATURAL REMEDIES

THE CONVENTIONAL MEDICAL VIEW

When Dr. Thurstan Brewin, FRCP, a cancer specialist, wrote an article for the Journal of the Royal Society of Medicine entitled: 'Logic and magic in mainstream and fringe medicine' (December 1993), he justified using the word 'fringe' for complementary, alternative, unconventional, natural and holistic by calling it 'a crisp monosyllable ... that its admirers were once happy to use'.

The writer is clearly not one of them. Yet he makes many valid points; not least, the reasons he suggests for the current boom in natural treatments. He first mentions the desire for more attention, more time, more sympathetic understanding, more hope. Next, the increasing wish of many patients to be given causes and explanations (even where none is really known or purely speculative). Thirdly, the desperate desire to try something different, especially in serious illness, accompanied by the need to feel 'in control'. Finally, he says, 'fringe medicine appeals to that side of our nature that dislikes logic and prefers magic – a basic instinct that may be seeking other outlets following a decline in religious observance'.

He also points out that 'mainstream' medicine honours the holistic principle, that of treating the whole person, not simply symptoms. Lord Joseph Lister, 1827–1912, one of the most important figures in the history of surgery, who introduced antiseptic techniques into the operating theatre, said that there was only one rule of good medical practice: 'put yourself in the patient's place'. Even more pertinently, Professor Sir William Osler,[1] commented that what matters is not what sort of disease the patient has, but what sort of patient has the disease.

What mainstream medics cannot swallow, and this is hardly surprising considering their (our) scientific training, is all this talk about the life force (e.g. the Chinese Ch'i, which acupuncture meridian lines are said to conduct); the rather vapid explanations therapists offer for every bodily ill; and the lack of properly controlled medical studies. Fringe practitioners and others claim

[1] (1849–1919), the Canadian medical educationalist whose book 'The Principles and Practice of Medicine' remained a standard medical work for years after its publication in 1892

that, for them, comparisons drawn from randomised pilot trials are not valid because of variations in treatment to suit the individual. (Homoeopathy is a case in point). But Dr. Brewin contradicts this. How can all benefits suddenly become invisible just because a formal comparison is made? Indeed, a constantly varying treatment policy can itself be legitimately compared with a more standardised policy. Alternatively, one particular aspect of a policy can be looked at to see whether it is doing good.

It isn't hard to see both points of view. Quite a few doctors practise complementary therapies, particularly osteopathy, chiropractic, acupuncture, homoeopathy and medical herbalism, although they don't necessarily accept the esoteric explanation of their modus operandi. Here I explain, from a medical perspective, some of the remedies with a substantial track record for relieving symptoms. Natural treatments for specific ailments are placed under their relevant chapters.

HERBAL MEDICINE

This underlies pharmaceutical practice the world over, and remains the major source of treatment in most underdeveloped countries. Many Western doctors take subsidiary courses in herbalism, and plant remedies are one of the most popular forms of complementary self-treatment in the UK and the US.

There are two views of how it works: medical doctors prescribe the remedies according to their chemical components' desired effects on whatever system of the body needs external aid: simple examples would be foxglove extract containing digitalis for heart failure, and senna pod tea for occasional constipation; the first slows down and strengthens the heart muscles, while the second stimulates the walls of the large bowel.

Holistic therapists stress the importance of the interaction between the energy fields of plants and humans, selecting herbal cures rather on the basis of boosting a person's life force, and combating stress and stale toxins in the tissues – two major 'holistic' causes of poor health.

Important points to remember about natural treatments, especially herbal medicines, is that if they work (which they do) they must have power (they have). They can therefore cause harm if used inappropriately. ALWAYS follow manufacturers' instructions and don't go rooting up wild herbs to treat yourself, unless you are one hundred per cent certain you can identify them correctly.

The herbs mentioned in the chapters of this book are an indication of names to look for when wishing to buy a herbal remedy from a chemist or health food shop; or names you may hear mentioned if you visit a medical herbalist for treatment. Always say what other treatments you are receiving (also tell the doctor if you are taking herbal or complementary medicines) as some remedies and medicines disagree with one another and can make you ill.

Don't take anything if you are pregnant unless prescribed by your doctor; and DON'T try to substitute a natural therapy, however good, for straightforward professional medical diagnosis and treatment for cancer, infections, or any other diseases that fail to respond to simple measures.

HOMOEOPATHIC MEDICINES

Nearly all of the above advice applies equally to homoeopathic treatments, except that these produce neither side effects nor unwanted symptoms. They are safe in the strengths in which you can buy them (from chemists, health shops etc.), and the worst really potent ones prescribed by a practitioner will do, is enhance some of the symptoms (or the ills that preceded these) that you are trying to get rid of.

You'll doubtless notice some of the horrid, even absurd, active constituents of the remedies – snake venom, arsenic etc.; but they are present in

149

extremely minute quantities – some really potent remedies are highly unlikely to contain even a trace of the original substance (all are of animal, plant or mineral origin). This is because the remedies are 'potentised' by grinding the original material into an inert carrier substance, e.g. lactose, in the case of tablets, and diluting them many times over. The beneficial effects therefore come, not from the active constituent itself, but from the electromagnetic imprint its molecules leave upon those of the carrier. An example would be Sepia, a cuttlefish extract used for depression and period pain, leaving its 'imprint' on lactose (milk sugar) and therefore able, when taken into the body, to correct energy imbalances connected to the symptoms which homoeopathists see as underlying health problems of all types.

The remedies are chosen according to the personality, physical type and individual (idiosyncratic) illness profile of particular patients, although the remedies available over the counter work at a basic symptom level as well. The underlying principle is that of 'like cures like', i.e. extremely small amounts of a substance will cure or relieve symptoms which larger amounts would bring on in a healthy person.

One example is Ipecachuana, used by medical doctors in ordinary amounts to induce vomiting, e.g. when a poisonous substance has been swallowed, tiny traces used in the homoeopathic remedy Ipecac are prescribed to relieve and cure nausea and vomiting.

AROMATHERAPY

Plant essences are used in today's most popular form of complementary therapy – massage – by both professional aromatherapists and masseurs, and for self treatment. They are too potent to be used alone, and the usual method is to add a few drops to a carrier oil such as sweet almond oil or corn oil. Other methods of administering aromatherapy essences include inhaling fumes after adding a few drops of the precious oils to steam; adding to bath water or water for hand- or foot-bathing; and evaporating them in a burner fuelled by a night-light for day or night time use. Some are sold as a cartridge which is inserted into the cigarette lighter of a car, to clear the atmosphere, aid concentration and ward off drowsiness.

ACUPUNCTURE

Acupuncture is the mainstay of Chinese medical practice, and involves a great deal of skill, both in knowing where along the body's meridians (invisible energy channels) to insert the acupuncture needles, and in identifying the energy blockage (the equivalent of a Western medical examination) beforehand. One major diagnostic aid is the pulse which, to Chinese acupuncturists, has a large number of qualities we in the West do not recognise; and from which much essential information can be obtained.

Acupuncture points small, discrete, high energy areas along the meridians in which the needles are stuck (or where pressure is applied, in acupressure), or smouldering herbs placed, in a technique called moxibustion. The understanding is that whatever method, attention paid to these minute regions unblocks the obstacle to the free energy flow (the Ch'i), restoring the natural, to body, mind and soul, and the person, therefore, to health. You may find acupuncture of use when lack of harmony seems to be part of your menstrual problem; typical examples are those that occur at times when the body's hormones are in a state of furore, such as PMS sufferers experience before periods, and during the menopause.

Now, for some products supported by research studies, you can buy to treat your own 'problem periods'.

HELPFUL PRODUCTS FOR PMS

1. MAGNESIUM OK.
Supplementary Magnesium. Since the scientist, Guy E. Abraham, first suggested (1983) magne-

sium deficiency as a cause of (many) PMS symptoms, anecdotal and professional experience has accumulated in support. Now, says the April 1992 issue of the *Journal of Sexual Medicine*, placebo-controlled studies in Pavia, Italy, have confirmed the help afforded by oral supplementary magnesium. Volunteers received 360 mg magnesium thrice daily from day 19 in their cycles until their next period. The magnesium content of cells rose, the supplements caused few side effects and the greatest benefit seemed to be reduction in irritability, tension, feelings of stress and depression.

We now know that magnesium works better in combination with other nutrients than as a single supplement. Its close association in the body with vitamin B6 (pyridoxine), for instance, has brought both to the forefront of PMS research. B6's sixty or so actions in the body include helping minerals cross the cell membrane (a highly complex, physico-chemical structure) from the fluid part of the blood (plasma) into the cells. (Abraham and his co-workers found that nine magnesium-deficient PMS sufferers who took 100 mg B6 twice daily for a month, had significantly higher plasma levels of magnesium, and *four times* as much magnesium in their red cells as those women who didn't take B6).

B6 also oversees the conversion of tryptophan and other amino acids into neurotransmitters (brain and nerve chemicals) that help to regulate mood and stabilise the stress response. Many claims have been made for it as a remedy for PMS tension and mood swings; but research teams have often reported disappointing results after administering it alone. Specialist J Kliejinen and his team, for example, whose paper 'Vitamin B6 in the treatment of premenstrual syndrome: a review' was published in the British Journal of Obstetrics and Gynaecology in 1990 (97:847–852), found that B6 was probably 'only mildly effective, if at all'.

Earlier (1989) in a Premenstrual Society 'PREMSOC' report of his own research findings: Dr. Michael Brush had spoken of the advantages of presenting vital nutrients such as magnesium in a multivitamin/mineral complex, 'which not only improves general nutritional levels but almost certainly has specific effects' – citing magnesium presented with, among others, zinc and several mainstream B vits such as B5, B2 and B1.

For his study, the results of which are shown below, Dr Brush selected Magnesium-OK from many available brands. It contains:

Vitamins: B1, B2, B6, C, D, E.
Minerals: Magnesium, Zinc, Potassium,
    Manganese, Selenium, Chromium, Copper.

Dr. Brush's Magnesium-OK Trial
(100 participants)
Better 69%
Variable 5%
No change 17%
Did not suit (due to yeast? colouring?) 7%
Pregnant 2%.

The recommended dose of Magnesium-OK is one tablet daily after meals without a break, but one twice daily from day 10 onwards, may be necessary when symptoms are severe. Never take more than four tablets because of the risk link between vitamin B6, gastric upsets and other theoretical conditions.

For the small minority of women sensitive to yeast and/or food colouring E. Magnesium-OK may not suit and yeastless Magnezie (Lifeplan Products Ltd.) is a possible alternative. Magnesium-OK must not be taken in conjunction with the anti-Parkinson drug L-dopa, and neither it nor any other kind of remedy or medication should be taken during pregnancy without the specific permission of a gynaecologist or GP. Magnesium OK is available from most health food shops and chemists in packs of 30 or 90 from £3.55

2. EVENING PRIMROSE OIL – THE FACTS FOR PROSTAGLANDIN SYNTHESIS.

Whole-foods encourage prostaglandin E1 production by eliminating dietary enemies and including cold-pressed polyunsaturates rich in essential fatty acid 'cis-linoleic acid' – the starter substance for making GLA (gammalinolenic acid) from which the cells synthesise prostaglandins E1.

You can be sure of getting your full GLA quota with Efamol evening primrose oil supplements. Efamol has been chosen for nearly every single evening primrose oil trial and clinical study, simply because research requires that the active ingredient(s) of a substance be reliably present in every sample at a guaranteed concentration and purity.

The Efamol Company employed world-ranking geneticists and plant specialists to collect and cross-breed different species of Oenothera biennis (evening primrose) until they had produced a plant whose seed oil fulfilled the exacting biochemical (and agricultural) conditions required. Research in this connection and in manufacture and purity control has been updated continuously over the past 20 years.

GLA, like many other organic compounds, can take a variety of molecular forms, and GLA in Efamol uniquely suits human and animal biochemistry. Optimal cell-friendliness, in turn, means optimal GLA digestion, absorption and utilisation.

Blackcurrant seeds, fungi and borage produce more GLA than evening primroses, but differences between their compatibilities with our needs, are very great. PMS sufferers use 500 mg Efamol capsules twice a day, the dose depending on symptom severity, i.e. from one to two capsules twice daily after food, to a maximum of six capsules twice daily, starting two days BEFORE symptoms appear. Efamol was criticised as a treatment for PMS because organisers of a double-blind cross-over trial in Sweden involving only 27 women reported in 1993, that no success could be attributed to Efamol because both placebo and treatment groups felt better and better as the study progressed. In other words, the placebo was so great it theoretically 'negated' Efamol's benefits.

It is unscientific to criticise Efamol's effectiveness in PMS on the strength of that one study; placebo response is often greater in illnesses with a strong psychological (which is not to imply imaginary) component.

Both atopic eczema and irritable bowel syndrome (IBS) tend to worsen in sufferers premenstrually; atopic eczema has been shown to respond exceptionally well to evening primrose oil GLA which has held a Product Licence from the

Committee on Safety of Medicines (CSM) to treat eczema under the name of Epogam for several years. (Evening primrose oil GLA is also prescribed on the NHS as Efamast for benign breast pain – mastalgia).

IBS causes abdominal pain, bloating, alternate diarrhoea and constipation, embarrassing bowel gas and frequent bowel upsets. In a double-blind placebo-controlled cross-over study in the US, involving 40 women with premenstrual worsening of these symptoms, none was helped by placebo whereas around 50% responded to Efamol: a statistically highly significant difference.

The first study of its kind, by Dr. Michael Brush at London's St. Thomas's Hospital, chose 68 PMS sufferers who had already failed to respond to at least one other treatment (and therefore would be less likely to show a placebo effect – transient improvement in symptoms due to psychological expectations rather than to the medicine). All the women took 4×500 mg Efamol twice daily, most starting three days before the expected start of symptoms and the rest with the worst symptoms taking Efamol throughout their cycles, with these findings:

Very marked improvement change	Partial relief	No
61%	23%	15%

There's also a special premenstrual PMP Pack – with Efavite tablets to take with the Efamol. Efavite contain vitamins C, B3 (niacin) and B6 (pyridoxine), plus zinc, co-factors in prostaglandin synthesis from GLA.

3. SUPPLEMENTARY MULTINUTRIENTS

The argument in favour of a daily multivitamin/ mineral combination for the whole population, from infants to centenarians, is beyond question from the point of view of preventive medicine; and is growing stronger weekly as national health service medical services become increasingly overtaxed and therefore inefficient.

The soundest way to develop an effective nutrient formulation is, first, to establish scientifically the relevance of particular vitamins and minerals to the disorder in question, and then to provide them in meaningful amounts, taking into account both positive and negative interactions. This avoids unnecessary "mega" doses, and the inclusion of nutrients that detract from one another's performance. The health product company Vitabiotics adopted this policy in creating Premence for premenstrual syndrome.

Premence contains 12 nutrients which act synergistically, i.e. their combined effect is greater than the sum of their individual effects.

Premence contains niacin (B3), pyridoxmine

(B6), vitamin C and zinc, all required for the utilisation of GLA (see 'evening primrose oil' above). Its other vitamins are: A (for healthy skin and mucous membranes, and to help correct hormone imbalance); thiamine (B1) and cyanocobalamin (B12), both important for a healthy nervous system - B12 also aids red cell manufacture; E, vital for the sex organs and fertility, and shown in clinical studies to aid PMS symptoms, especially breast tenderness; and folic acid, for healthy ovaries and blood cells.

In addition to zinc, Premence's minerals and trace elements include magnesium, iodine and iron. Magnesium is an antioxidant, and combats stress; supplementary magnesium corrects deficiency of this mineral associated with a low level of brain opamine which can cause nervous tension and anxiety. Iodine is vital to the thyroid gland, which regulates the metabolic rate (rate at which we burn food fuel); the iron reduces the risk of iron deficiency anaemia, encourages the development of new red cells and promotes oxygen transport and energy production.

One study of Premence's effects on PMS, involved 78 sufferers aged 24-45 years with moderate to severe symptoms but no other gynaecological disorders, who were not on oral contraceptives or HRT, and not suffering from cancer, diabetes or epilepsy. Forty-three of the women took

Premence and the rest, a dummy placebo, the results being compared by both questionnaires for the pre- and postmenstrual cycle phases, and after the study, by self assessment. 72.1% said their symptoms had improved a lot. 18.6% had noticed a slight improvement and 9.5% no improvement.

HELPFUL PRODUCTS FOR MENOPAUSAL SYMPTOMS

MELBROSIA PLD

Melbrosia pld (pour les dames – for women) from Austria, is a health food supplement of natural substances for the relief of menopausal symptoms. Extensive medical trials by doctors and consultant gynaecologists have revealed similar benefits to those of HRT, but without side effects or the need for 'top-up' conventional treatment. It contains bee-collected flower pollen, fermented pollen (also called bee bread or perga), royal jelly and vitamin C.

Melbrosia studies have been carried out in most European countries. I will report one by Professor Francesco Corletto, a Venetian medical specialist and expert in complementary therapies, in detail. His paper published in May 1993, discussed a trial involving two groups each of 26 women aged 45–54, with menopausal discomfort. Physical

161

symptoms included hot flushes and sweats, lethargy, insomnia, a racing heartbeat and headaches; psychological ones ranged from poor memory and concentration, tension and mental fatigue to reduced sex drive, anxiety and depression.

The women themselves gave a scale value to their symptoms, while doctors similarly assessed their racing heart beat and insomnia producing a total (global) value for each of the two groups. Examinations and assessments were carried out before and after the six month trial period, during which each of the 52 participants took three capsules daily – half of them Melbrosia pld, the other half identical dummies or placebos. None took any other medicines at all, (the necessity to do so, simply resulted in disqualification from the study).

Results: there were no reported side effects. Women taking placebo capsules showed no significant improvement in their symptoms. The Melbrosia pld group experienced significant symptom relief.

Another trial by Professor Corletto assessed the effects of Melbrosia pld on blood fats (as mentioned in this book elsewhere, heart attack risks in women rise after the age of 55 to exceed men's, because reduced oestrogen production adversely affects cholesterol and triglyceride blood levels). Lipid levels were assessed before and after the 12 month treatment period, during which the women took three Melbrosia pld capsules a day. None had had HRT or any other treatment that could affect blood fat metabolism, within a year of the start of the trial. The final analysis showed that Melbrosia pld helps to re-establish a balanced blood fat profile as effectively as HRT, but without side effects.

Pollen, Melbrosia's main constituent, has been analysed by many research workers since the 1940s. Its complete formulation has still not been fully documented, but it is known to contain around 12% water, 20% protein, 30% free amino acids (protein building blocks), and 30% 'other nutrients', including carbohydrates, unsaturated fatty acids, plant hormones, minerals, vitamins and trace elements, which are minerals such as zinc and copper required in very small amounts.

Pollen *proteins* include enzymes and co-enzymes (biological catalysts that trigger and oversee vital cellular processes), especially ones like adenosine triphosphate and cytochrome C, involved with energy production; and ample supplies of the genetic nucleic acids DNA and RNA. Its minerals and trace elements include sodium, potassium, magnesium, calcium, iron, copper, zinc, manganese, silica, phosphorous, chlorine and sulphur. Pollen's most important vitamins are beta carotene (provitamin A), B1 (thiamin), C, D, E and K.

Pollen may also be the world's richest natural source of *bioflavonoids*. Found combined with naturally occurring vitamin C, these compounds are powerful antioxidants, which means that they mop up and thereby neutralise free radicals. An excess of these highly charged and unstable atoms, released by the cells normal processes, help to cause degenerative disorders such as arthritis, wrinkled skin and early ageing, and also cancer.

Pollen's main bioflavonoid, rutin, strengthens and controls capillaries, minute vessels which, in the skin, are closely involved with the rushes of blood that help to cause menopausal hot flushes and sweats. Bioflavonoids are widely used as a dietary supplement, alone or as part of a larger nutrient complex; and oxerutins are prescribed as the drug Paroven by doctors for waterlogged tissues in the lower legs, when inefficient e.g. varicose veins are failing to transport blood up the body against the force of gravity, and producing a back pressure. Bioflavonoids also benefit the circulation as a whole; act as a diuretic against fluid retention and bloating; encourage the production of bile by the gall bladder (which aids fat digestion); and help to balance the actions of the thymus, adrenals, pancreas and thyroid gland.

Vitamin C is the antistress vitamin, and a powerful antioxidant. *Royal jelly*, on which the highly fertile queen feeds throughout her long life (compared with other bees), is manufactured as a thick, creamy substance by the workers in special glands in their heads. Basically, it is a compound of pollen loosely bound with water, containing a biogenic stimulator called 50-hydroxy-decen-acid which promotes healthy cell growth and renewal. Like pollen, its complete formulation has not yet been determined. *Bee bread* is formed from pollen packed into waxen cells and allowed to ferment at its own pace in the warm, dark, humid atmosphere of the hive. Its constituents are roughly those of unfermented pollen, but they're at least 50% more bioavailable (accessible to the body). Melbrosia plc also combats osteoporosis; but I want to talk about another supplement, developed in the UK, for use in this condition.

2. EFECAL

This dietary supplement combines calcium and two essential fatty acids to combat osteoporosis which, as we saw in the previous chapter, is one of the health hazards of the post-menstrual years. Dr. Brenda Reynolds, research adviser to Efecal's manufacturers, Efamol Ltd., adds the information that 100,000 men (and 2 million women) have osteoporosis in the UK alone, 'although only around 76,000 patients receive any related treatment'. More women than men suffer because loss of oestrogen at the menopause predisposes so strongly to bone demineralisation, but factors affecting both sexes include poor diet, lack of sunlight (needed to make vitamin D in the skin), alcohol, smoking and too little weight-bearing exercise.

As Dr. Reynolds goes on to say: 'More than one in five orthopaedic beds in hospitals are used by osteoporosis-related fracture patients... up to one in five hip fracture patients die shortly after injury whilst more than half become dependent on others. A major osteoporosis conference reported that in 1990 in the UK, 46,000 fractured femurs cost £165 million for acute care and resulted in a mortality figure of 15%'.

The hormone calcitonin from the parathyroid glands in the neck, which helps to regulate the body's use of calcium, and vitamin D, HRT, steroids, sodium fluoride, biphosphonates (the element phosphorus is a major component of bones and supplementary calcium) are used medically to try to prevent osteoporosis. They all work up to a point, but none is entirely satisfactory.

Prostaglandins (PGs), the hormone-like cell chemicals discussed earlier in connection with PMS, are also important for strong, healthy bones. A group called PGE 2s encourage the skeleton to leach out calcium. PGE 2s are formed from the essential fatty acid arachidonic acid,

166

made in the body and found in red meat. The PMS-combatting PGE 1s (see Chapter 7) have the opposite effect, and strengthen bones. PGE 1s are made in the body from gammalinolenic acid (GLA). GLA is formed in the body from cis-linoleic acid in polyunsaturated plant oils, and found reformed in breast milk and evening primrose oil.

A third group, PG E3s, have a healthy effect like the PGE 1s. They come from a fatty acid called eicosapentaenoic acid (EPA), another vital nutrient made in the body from *alpha*linolenic acid found in plants, together with DHA (doco-hexapentaenoic acid), the vital brain cell nutrient. Both EPA and DHA are also found in fish oils. The presence of large doses of alpha-linolenic acid, EPA and DHA also conveniently minimises the amount of any arachidonic acid present.

The production of PGE 1s and 3s from GLA and EPA is reduced by many factors; most pertinently in middle and old age, the ageing process itself, and poor diet. Ageing is a dual risk factor because it retards the formation of new bone (and other tissues), and discourages PGE 1 conversion from gammalinolenic acid (GLA). Similarly, the high blood sugar levels found in diabetes discourage helpful prostaglandin production, and can also trigger osteoporosis by increasing the loss of calcium in urine.

The balance between the PGEs 1 and 3, on the one hand, and of PGE 2 on the other, is, therefore, crucial; and it is directly related to the levels of the essential fatty acids (EFAs) in the body from which these prostaglandins are made. We cannot take prostaglandins to help prevent or treat osteoporosis or any other complaint, because they are chemically delicate and short-lived (PGs are made 'on site' wherever they're needed in the body, and immediately destroyed when they have done their work).

We can, however, eat the green leafy vegetables and polyunsaturates that provide cis-linoleic acid and alphalinolenic acid, to aid the manufacture of GLA and EPA; *and* take GLA and EPA as supplements, to compensate for any difficulty we may have in using them. A normal diet should contain 4–6% essential fatty acids, especially the average Western diet which is high in saturated fat (which also intereferes with PG production). Besides favouring prostaglandin manufacture, dietary EPAs keep cell membranes fluid and flexible, lower blood fat levels (large doses of fish oil raise blood levels of protective LDL cholesterol), and enhance calcium absorption and the utilization of vitamin D.

Research – laboratory and human clinical studies have shown that the relationship between EFAs, trostaglandins and calcium in bone metabolism can be exploited to help prevent and treat osteoporosis.

A paper in a 1993 issue of the Journal of Urology, described how urology specialist Mr. A C Buck and his team in Scotland had given 30 patients with recurrent calcium urinary stones, 6g daily of fish oil (FO), evening primrose oil (EPO) or sunflower oil each for 12 weeks, after first stopping all treatment and stabilising them on a standard calcium diet of 800 mg daily. All treatment increased calcium absorption from the intestine, but EPO and FO increased it most of all. (Sunflower oil is a polyunsaturate containing cis-linoleic acid). Calcium excretion in the urine was also substantially reduced in the FO and EPO/FO groups, independently of gut absorption; and the calcium content of bone was significantly increased.

The same team also gave laboratory rats FO, EPO, FO/EPO combined, or sunflower oil, before and while they were being treated with calcium gluconate to try and make them develop urinary stones. The loss of calcium in the urine was significantly reduced, especially the EPO and EPO/FO groups who formed no stones whatever.

Meanwhile, in South Africa, patients with osteoporosis confirmed by bone densitometry, received supplementary EPO, FO, EPO/FO or olive oil placebo for 16 weeks, after which tests confirmed a decrease in the urinary loss of calcium (D H van Paperdorp and co-workers). Other studies have confirmed all these findings.

CONFIANCE

The usefulness of multiminerals in the relief of menopausal symptoms has been confirmed so many times by thousands of women that it is surprising that no pharmaceutical company has as yet worked out and tested its own formula, and applied for a licence to position their product on the prescription list.

Confiance was formulated to relieve and, hopefully, prevent some of the menopausal symptoms caused by the (relative) malnutrition from which many women suffer, when middle-age and low oestrogen levels raise their baseline nutritional needs. It works; I've recommended it to dozens of women patients and friends, and it costs £4.25 for a month's supply (30 tablets), or £10.45 for 80 from Boots, Holland and Barrett, other good chemists and health stores. Here's what a single tablet supplies.

Magnesium	175 mg
Manganese	2 mg
Boron	1 mg
Selenium	25 mcg (micrograms)
Chromium	25 mcg
Vitamin B1	5 mg
Vitamin B2	5 mg

Vitamin B3   10 mg
Vitamin B6   50 mg
Vitamin E   200 i.u. (international units)

Confiance study: here are some details of a Confiance study involving 200 volunteers enlisted through regional advertising, 124 (62%) of whom returned completed questionnaires as arranged, after taking one Confiance tablet daily for 90 days. Funded by the manufacturers, the results were independently monitored by medical statisticians.

The women experienced an average of more than seven symptoms, for just under four (3.92) years. Each woman had to categorise her symptoms at the start of the study as 'severe', 'slight' or 'occasional'; or 'not a problem'; and indicate at the end of the three months on Confiance whether her symptoms were worse, the same or better. Twenty-seven and a half (per cent) had no problems before treatment; 38% had slight or occasional symptoms and 33.5% suffered severely (the rest didn't reply). Here is the list of symptoms:
(1) hot flushes
(2) cold sweats
(3) headaches
(4) weight gain
(5) insomnia
(6) depression
(7) lack of incentive

(8) lack of confidence
(9) palpitations
(10) poor concentration

Hot flushes were the commonest symptom (85%), and weight gain was ranked as 'severe' by 48% of the total. A volunteer who did not have a particular symptom before starting on Confiance could only remain the same or deteriorate after treatment; only one out of 256 symptom responses showed this. 65% of the responses describing symptoms as severe showed an improvement with treatment, 31% remained the same, 2% deteriorated and 2% did not reply. Responses referring to slight or occasional symptoms before treatment, indicated that 53% improved on Confiance, 41% stayed the same, 2% deteriorated and 4% didn't reply.

Excepting weight gain (41%) and lack of incentive (47%), the majority of the volunteers with severe symptoms improved with treatment. Symptoms most effectively relieved by Confiance included cold sweats (91%), headaches (81%), and hot flushes (80%).

Women with slight or occasional symptoms responded less well to treatment.

The symptoms that were best relieved in this group were cold sweats (70%), palpitations (85%) and hot flushes (83%). Weight gain (32%),

172

insomnia (35%) and lack of incentive (43%) improved least of all.

The severity of the symptoms as classified by the volunteers in this study was, of course subjective, so the effect of treatment on specific symptoms, regardless of severity, was determined as well. Apart from weight gain and insomnia (both 37.5%), all other symptoms showed a greater than 50% response to Confiance:

Cold sweats (78.5%) and hot flushes (74.5%) showed the greatest response to treatment.

80% of the women (4 out of every five volunteers) indicated that they would purchase Confiance in the future).

A HELP FOR ALMOST ALL PERIOD PROBLEMS – CHLORELLA

WHAT IS CHLORELLA?

A single-celled alga (primitive plant) about the size of a red blood cell, is one of the oldest life forms known, one that fossil evidence shows has existed for around 2.5 billion years. Discovered in 1890, it is now known to be a naturally occurring, multinutrient wholefood, and probably one of the first links in the food chain, helping to transform the earth's original toxic atmosphere into a life-supporting, green environment.

So called because of its high chlorophyll content, Chlorella is found in fresh water rivers and ponds, and has been extensively studied since the 1850s, especially in Japan where it is the most popular health supplement, and where the government have designated it a 'functional food', a food that may have medical and healing qualities. It is taken in larger quantities than most dietary nutrients (e.g. 12 tablets or 3 grams loose powder, which can be added to drinks, soups, casseroles and other dishes).

My interest in Chlorella stems from my experience of the energy boost it can provide: the Aston Villa team take Chlorella daily to boost stamina; it's the most popular functional food/health supplement in Japan; and in the US, NASA are researching it as a source of food for astronauts. It also helps to prevent and relieve a wide range of health problems, including some associated with Problem Periods.

Chlorella is rich in protein (60%), and in free amino acids (protein building blocks); in fact, it contains three times as much protein as beef, and can produce protein fifty times more efficiently than other protein plant crops such as soya beans. It's rich in fibre and complex carbohydrates (20%); yet contains only 11% fat, 82% of which is the polyunsaturated (healthy) type.

Chlorella also supplies over 20 vitamins and

minerals, including beta carotene, B complex, vitamin C with bioflavonoids, iron, zinc, selenium, and calcium and magnesium in the optimal forms (and proportions) for integration into the skeleton. And is a unique source of vitamin B12 (cyanocobalamin), vital for a healthy nervous system and foetal growth, and often dangerously low or even absent from the diets of vegetarians and vegans since it is largely concentrated in animal-derived foods and related products.

2. USES – WHAT IT CAN DO FOR YOU

Its special relevance in this book is threefold: firstly, it enhances the oxygen-carrying power of the blood; secondly, it helps to minimise free radical damage; lastly, Chlorella may be of benefit to you if you have menstrual problems other than those falling into the first two categories.

(1) The high chlorophyll content of Chlorella (the richest known source of this green plant pigment) helps to build the red blood cells (vital if you suffer from anaemia, heavy periods or non-menstrual bleeding). Chlorophyll itself can be converted into haemoglobin, the oxygen-transporting pigment in human and most animal blood. It is also a powerful detoxifier, aiding the elimination of waste materials as well as combating the effects of environmental and other pollutants. Chlorella also

enhances the functions of the liver, one of which is the removal and destruction of ageing red cells, and the conservation of their haemoglobin and iron for future use.

Oxygen is essential for all life functions, and for vitality, energy, a sense of well being, and a natural resistance to infections and other diseases. Chlorella's unique CGF (Chlorella Growth Factor) which enhances natural growth processes in cultures of single-celled plants and animals, doubtless helps to account for the energy boost derived from daily helpings of Chlorella. CGF has not yet been fully analysed, but it is thought to be a sort of nucleopeptide (similar to the structures in genetic DNA and RNA), but containing sulphur.

(2) All of Chlorella's vitamins, minerals and trace elements are antioxidants and, since free radicals have been implicated in malignant cellular changes, women may benefit from a degree of protection against reproductive organ cancers. In the laboratory, in fact, Chlorella extract has been shown to reduce the rate of sarcoma (muscle) tumour growth in mice by almost 53% over 25 days; and also to encourage the release of *interferon*, a product of the immune defence cells with powerful anti-tumour growth effects.

Antioxidant nutrients also stimulate the immune defence cells, needed to be especially alert and potent to deal with infective organisms.

So Chlorella may well be of overall benefit if you are prone to *vaginal infections* or *pelvic inflammatory disease*.

(3) Other specific uses: Chlorella encourages wounds to heal and may be of use after an operation or if you are suffering from a cervical erosion. The particular combinations of essential fatty acids and calcium, magnesium and phosphorus encourage the remineralisation of bones and help to guard against *osteoporosis*. And a study in Japan involving women aged 45–55, when compared with similar, age-matched women taking a dummy placebo, found that Chlorella especially relieved constipation, alterations in temperature and fatigue, among the 18 menopausal symptoms tested.

3. TAKING YOUR CHLORELLA

If you're wondering whether you could ever face daily doses of green pond slime, though it were to ensure a healthy and prosperous life for the next five decades, I should mention that the algae used in Chlorella Health tablets are cultivated in pure mineral water under conditions monitored by a team of microbiologists. After they have been harvested, Chlorella is then spray-dried and packaged as powder, or compressed into tablets, nothing being either added or taken away.

The finished product has a mild, nutty flavour similar to raw peanuts; this can easily be disguised by swallowing the tablets or powder whole with water or fruit juice, or simply mixing the powder into other foods, as already mentioned.

Green pond slime, therefore, although providing an excellent lead line for health journalists when Chlorella first attracted UK media attention, is as far removed from what you actually see and take, as the raw, dripping pancreas and thymus gland of a recently slaughtered lamb or calf is from a French restaurant entrée of sweetbreads cooked in Cognac and cream.

Chlorella costs around £9.00 for one month's supply, from Boots (by order only), other chemists, Holland and Barrett and all good health food shops or by mail order from the distributors: Chlorella Health Ltd, 4th Floor, Russell Chambers, Covent Garden, London WC2E 8AA, tel.: 071 240-4775.

INDEX

A

Acupuncture: 151–152
Adhesions: 40, 42
Amarant Trust: 135
Anaemia, iron deficiency: 43, 48, 126
Androgens: 24
Anorexia: 25
Anticoagulants: 54–55, 126
Antidepressants: 20
Antidiarrhoea drugs: 55
Antinauseant drugs: 55
Antispasmodics: 55
Aphrodisiacs: 14
Aromatherapy: 151
Austria: 161

B

Bee bread: see Perga.
Bernard, Claude: 15–16
Bioflavonoids: 164
Bleeding, dysfunctional: 62–66
  and drugs: 66
  and hormones: 63–64
  and obesity: 65–66
  and weight loss, sudden: 64–65
  heavy: see Menorrhagia.
  irregular: 12, 60–68, 126
  menstrual: 6, 7, 10

  non-menstrual: 69–81
  post-coital (i.e. after intercourse): 61, 70, 74
Blood pressure: 2–3
Brewin, Thurston Dr.: 145–147

C

Calcium: 113, 165
Cancer, and women: 69–70
  of the cervix: 75–81; causes: 78–79; stages: 77–78
  survival rates: 81; treatment: 80
  of the ovaries: 117–119, 127
  of the uterus: 116–117
Characteristics, sexual: 23–24
Cheese effect: 20,
Ch'i: 146, 152
Chlorella: 173–178
Chlorophyll: 175, 176
Colposcopy: 80
COMA: 92
Corletto, Francesco: 162–163
Corpus luteum: 9
Cysts, ovarian: 8–9. See also Ovaries, Polycystic.

179